Hormone Therapy

Katherine Sherif

Hormone Therapy

A Clinical Handbook

Foreword by Morris Notelovitz

Springer

Katherine Sherif, MD, FACP
Drexel Center for Women's Health
Drexel University College of Medicine
Philadelphia, PA, USA

ISBN 978-1-4614-6267-5 ISBN 978-1-4614-6268-2 (eBook)
DOI 10.1007/978-1-4614-6268-2
Springer New York Heidelberg Dordrecht London

Library of Congress Control Number: 2013933360

Printed on acid-free paper

Springer is part of Springer Science+Business Media (www.springer.com)

To My Parents
Frances, Fawzy & Amal

Foreword

Aging is universal, as are the physiological shifts that come with the body's diminished estrogen production in the perimenopausal years. Estrogen is not just a sex steroid. Estrogen receptors are present in every tissue and organ system, and the hormone is an essential component of vital health and wellness for all women. Estrogen is never depleted, only deficient; for many women, its components estrone and estradiol need to be monitored to support a woman's best physical and mental functionality.

What the best health professionals treating women for estrogen replacement, replenishment, and maintenance know is that the only pharmacologic approach to replicating the premenopausal estradiol milieu is via transdermal therapy. They also know that individuation of therapy is key. This means tailoring therapy according to an individual woman's clinical needs and her age, with a progressive downward adjustment of dosage over time.

Estrogen and all hormone therapy treatments are complementary to the other health measures of proper exercise and nutrition, and to certain disease-specific medications. Over many years of practice, I have learned that this kind of therapy is not a panacea for all women, but that on an annual basis, women should be asked this set of questions: "If you are taking hormone therapy, why? And if not, why not?"

Boca Raton, FL, USA — Morris Notelovitz, M.D., Ph.D

About Dr. Notelovitz

Dr. Morris Notelovitz, M.D., Ph.D., is a Board Certified gynecologist and Fellow of both the American and the Royal Colleges of Obstetrics and Gynecology. He has served in senior academic positions and in private practice both in South Africa and in the United States.

He is the founder of the Adult Women's Health Alliance, a nonprofit multidisciplinary consortium of national healthcare organizations. Based on the clinical application of validated science, the mission of the Alliance is the promotion of health and the prevention of disease in adult women.

Dr. Notelovitz has authored over 280 articles, chapters, and abstracts on adult women's health issues and four books for the lay public and has co-edited five books for physicians. He is a Consultant in Adult Women's Health and Medicine, is President of the Adult Women's Health Alliance, and is Chief Scientific Officer of Cognifem, LLC, a company based on predictive medicine and preventive therapeutics.

Preface

When it comes to the menopausal transition, and whether it's perimenopause that can begin as early as 35, or postmenopause, some women experience very few symptoms. Other women, unfortunately, experience many symptoms, some severe, that interfere with their ability to lead a happy and productive life. For decades when it came to treating the symptoms of menopause, women were treated as a homogenous population. The menopausal transition was defined as an "estrogen deficiency disease" to be fixed with "estrogen". The role of progesterone and testosterone was ignored. Not only was estrogen (mostly one oral formulation) prescribed for symptoms, but doctors exhorted asymptomatic women to take it for this deficiency state. There was no careful discussion about individual symptoms and treatment possibilities—little monitoring and follow-up, and little understanding of perimenopause.

Things have changed. Hormone therapy can no longer be expected to be the "cure" for aging that clinicians only a few years ago desired it to be. We no longer expect it to decrease the risk of heart disease, in fact, in certain formulations and within certain subgroups, it may increase risks for breast cancer and heart disease. Today, HT used as menopause management focuses on a woman's specific and individual symptoms. It pays close attention to what a patient reports. It understands the science behind hormone replacement.

Women's health, menopause, and hormone therapy are hot-button topics. Because of this, clinicians need to help our patients demystify the confusing popular reports about menopause and about hormone therapies, and we need to be able to understand the popular remedies and information that are readily available, and which our patients may bring to our attention, seeking medical guidance.

The range of menopause years, from perimenopause to post-menopause, offer us a window of therapeutic opportunity, in which clinicians can help women move from their years of reproductive possibility, into the post-menopausal period, in the healthiest ways possible. This clinical handbook includes directions for prescribing HT in the safest and most effective ways possible.

This handbook aims to give clinicians—whether Physicians, Nurse Practitioners, Physician's Assistants, residents in the fields of Internal Medicine, Gynecology and Family Medicine, and others—the specific information they need to prescribe Hormone Therapy/Hormone Replacement Therapy.

Hormone Therapy offers a depth and breadth of practical prescribing experience, combined with an understanding of the basic science and clinical studies.

This handbook emerges from many years of research experience and clinical practice. Menopause, retrospectively defined as beginning 12 months after the last menstrual period (LMP), occurs at the mean age of 51.3 years. However, the transition into menopause, defined as perimenopause, may be associated with symptoms as early as 35, and for many women, may persist for years beyond the LMP. Menopause is characterized by low serum concentrations of estrogen, progesterone, and androgen steroids. By contrast, in the perimenopausal years serum steroids are far less predictable within individuals. For that reason, the use of follicle stimulating hormone (FSH) to predict reproductive stage is imprecise. As a corollary, hormonal therapy to alleviate perimenopausal symptoms is not necessarily the same for symptoms that persist after menopause. Additionally, several hundred thousand women undergo abrupt menopause due to oophorectomy, chemotherapeutic agents (including oral medications), and less commonly, autoimmune disease. In 2012, the cohort of women between the ages of 40 and 60 years who may be symptomatic is roughly 44 million.

This is essentially and foremost a prescription handbook. Busy clinicians looking for ways to prescribe HT for varying symptoms of perimenopause and menopause should turn directly to Part II: Prescription of HT.

HT has had such a controversial history over the course of the twentieth century and into the twenty-first. This handbook demystifies the controversial studies that have grabbed media headlines and provide a larger context for safe and effective use. I hope that clinicians will use this handbook and the information herein to more confidently prescribe, and to educate their patients. The treatment of perimenopausal and menopausal symptoms has had several iterations. Much of the confusion arises from the simplistic view that the entire menopausal transition is an "estrogen" (as a general term distinct from estradiol, estrone, and estriol) deficiency (irrelevant of progesterone), that it is uniform and lends itself to uniform treatment. The significance of various types of estrogens, progesterone, and testosterone, as well as their prohormones and derivatives, and new knowledge about steroid receptors present in all tissues (and not just the reproductive organs) will help clinicians and women fine tune treatment for the best possible outcomes.

What this clinical handbook offers is the up-to-date usage guidelines for understanding women's menopause symptoms, and prescribing HT as relief, in ways that present the least risk and the best efficacy and outcome for women patients. Because HT has been controversial, however, many clinicians are unsure of what to make of the relative risks and benefits of HT, and where the most current research and clinical practice stands. In addition, our patients often have a fairly sophisticated engagement with the media headlines around HT use and often ask their doctors to explain this to them so that they can feel more comfortable with an HT prescription that when done transdermally, can safely relieve their severe menopause symptoms. That is why unlike some other handbooks, a history of the prescription, studies, and cultural shifts around HT use has been included, in Part IV.

Philadelphia, PA, USA Katherine Sherif, MD, FACP

About Dr. Sherif

The author, Dr. Katherine Sherif, is Chief of Clinical Programs in Women's Health, and Director, Drexel Center for Women's Health. She is also Associate Professor in the Department of Medicine, Drexel University College of Medicine. She is the co-editor of *Women's Health in Clinical Practice: A Handbook for Primary Care* (2008) and a member of the Writing Group of the *American Heart Association* (2007 and 2011) "Guidelines for Cardiovascular Disease Prevention in Women." Her clinical practice focuses on menopause and general women's health. She is the cofounder and director of the nation's first academic Center for Polycystic Ovary Syndrome, established in 2000.

Contents

Part I
Managing Perimenopausal and Postmenopausal Symptoms with the New Menopausal HT

1. FAQ: Definitions of Menopause and Biological Actions of Sex Steroids

Keywords Menopause • Menopause age • Perimenopause • Bioidentical hormone replacement • Estrogen

Introduction

There has been great confusion about the name of this stage of women's health and reproductive lives, with vagueness to the term menopause, and the introduction of the stage of perimenopause, or premenopause, as something that doctors, and women, are starting to understand on its own. It is helpful to divide menopause into the stages of perimenopause and postmenopause, as women may experience different symptoms during these times, and clinicians may prescribe differently, based on symptoms and on the results of clinical studies and trials of HT efficacy and safety.

Use the definition of reproductive stages from the Stages of Reproductive Aging Workshop STRAW + 10 (definition of reproductive stages), updated in 2012. See Fig. 1.1. STRAW identifies ten stages of ovarian aging based upon pattern of menstrual cycles. STRAW may help identify where women are on the reproductive spectrum and may be used to help individualize therapy. STRAW was developed as a research tool (Harlow SD et al. JCEM 2012: 1159–1168). For the sake of simplicity, the phrase "menopausal symptoms" will be used to refer to symptoms that occur during perimenopause and menopause.

Q. What is premenopause?

A. Premenopause encompasses the time period from menarche to the onset of variable menstrual intervals (≥7 days difference in intervals) which corresponds to mid-to-late thirties and early fourties.

K. Sherif, *Hormone Therapy: A Clinical Handbook*,
DOI 10.1007/978-1-4614-6268-2_1,

Menarche (at stage −5) FMP (0) (between stages −1 and +1a)

Stage	-5	-4	-3b	-3a	-2	-1	+1 a	+1b	+1c	+2
Terminology	**REPRODUCTIVE**				**MENOPAUSAL TRANSITION**		**POSTMENOPAUSE**			
	Early	Peak	Late		Early	Late	Early			Late
					Perimenopause					
Duration	*variable*				*variable*	1-3 years	2 years (1+1)		3-6 years	*Remaining lifespan*
PRINCIPAL CRITERIA										
Menstrual Cycle	Variable to regular	Regular	Regular	Subtle changes in Flow/ Length	*Variable Length* Persistent ≥7-day difference in length of consecutive cycles	Interval of amenorrhea of >=60 days				
SUPPORTIVE CRITERIA										
Endocrine FSH AMH Inhibin B			Low Low	Variable* Low Low	↑ Variable* Low Low	↑ >25 IU/L** Low Low	↑ Variable Low Low		Stabilizes Very Low Very Low	
Antral Follicle Count			Low	Low	Low	Low	Very Low		Very Low	
DESCRIPTIVE CHARACTERISTICS										
Symptoms						Vasomotor symptoms *Likely*	Vasomotor symptoms *Most Likely*			*Increasing* symptoms of urogenital atrophy

* Blood draw on cycle days 2-5 ↑ = elevated

**Approximate expected level based on assays using current international pituitary standard[67-69]

Fig. 1.1. The STRAW definitions of reproductive stages, 2012 update.

Q. What is perimenopause?

A. The onset of variable cycle intervals signals the menopausal transition and is defined as "perimenopause." In early perimenopause, menstrual cycle intervals may vary ≥7 days in women with previously regular cycles. Perimenopause is characterized by a gradual decline in progesterone production, concomitant with various fluctuations in estradiol. Not only are absolute levels of progesterone decreased, but the ratios of estradiol to progesterone and estrone to estradiol are altered. Women in perimenopause are those most likely to seek treatment for symptoms. While early perimenopause includes cycles that vary by more than 7 days, late perimenopause includes ≥2 months of amenorrhea.

In Fig. 1.2 the SWAN investigators (2012) concluded that based upon a large population of women (n=1,316), estradiol levels in the perimenopausal years fell into one of four patterns.

- The first was a slow decline of estradiol, mirroring the slow decline of progesterone (26.9 %)—a pattern seen mostly in Chinese and Japanese women.
- The second pattern was flat—this pattern was seen predominantly in obese women (body mass index >30) (28.6 %).

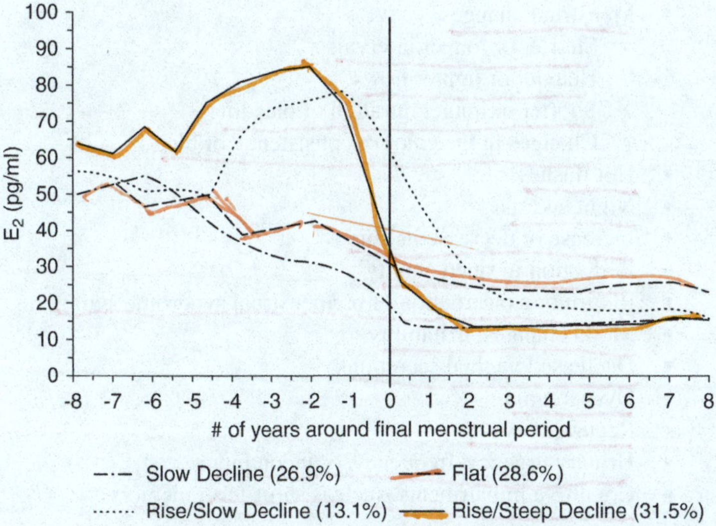

Fig. 1.2. Trajectory of E_2 across the FMP. Significant predictors for trajectory separation were race/ethnicity and BMI (see supplemental Table 2 for modeling details). E_2 levels were the average observed serum E_2 levels at each time point. Time-varying age, SHBG, and cycle day of blood draw were adjusted in the model. The model accuracy diagnostics showed that the capacity of the model to separate women among the groups was good. The AvePP ranged from 0.72 to 0.81 and the OCC ranged from 6.44 to 10.98 [30].

- The third pattern is described as a rise and slow decline (13.1 %), most likely to be seen in Chinese women and overweight women (BMI 25–30).
- The fourth pattern is a rise in estradiol levels 4–5 years preceding the LMP with a steep decline beginning one year prior to the LMP (31.5 %) most likely seen in normal weight (BMI <25) White and Black women.

In perimenopause, women still have monthly menstrual periods despite fluctuating estradiol and abrupt changes in hormone ratios. Progesterone, on average, begins a slow decline at age 35 years, while in the most symptomatic group, estradiol rises rapidly and has superimposed erratic surges. Testosterone steadily decreases. There is also hypothalamic-pituitary-ovarian resistance to the feedback cycle. There may be ovulatory cycles, anovulatory cycles, and/or estradiol surges during the luteal phase. Symptoms may include

- Menstrual changes
  - Shorter or longer intervals
  - Heavier or lighter flows
  - Shorter or longer duration of bleeding
  - Changes in the color or consistency of blood
- Hot flushes
- Night sweats
- Increase or decrease in libido
- Reduction in sleep quality
- Return or exacerbation of premenstrual syndrome symptoms
- Mood changes, irritability
- Decreased vaginal secretions
- Dyspareunia
- Recurrent cystitis
- Urinary urgency, frequency, or incontinence
- Cognitive impairments, such as short-term memory

This period, lasting until a year after the total cessation of periods, is perimenopause. In the past, this has been called premenopause or menopause itself; the nomenclature has been confusing. The late perimenopausal transition to amenorrhea (cessation of periods) is much longer than had been thought and can last 2–8 years. Some women are symptomatic for as long as 15 years.

Q. What is menopause?

A. Menopause is the time period that begins after cessation of menstrual bleeding for 12 consecutive months. At this time, estradiol, progesterone, and testosterone production are low but present. A reduction in sex hormones due to diminishing ovarian reserve eventually results in the cessation of bleeding. Ovaries continue to produce hormones, though. Adrenal and adipocyte production of sex hormones become more prominent. Because there are estrogen and other sex hormone receptors in all tissues, not just the reproductive organs, menopause yields effects throughout all organ systems. Menopause is also called climacteric, especially in Europe.

Q. What is the time of actual menopause?

A. In clinical terms, actual menopause is defined as 12 consecutive months after the last menstrual period (LMP). The average age (for women in the United States) is 51.3 years. The age range for women to reach menopause is 38–55.

Q. What is Postmenopause?

A. For clarity, we use the term "menopause" instead of "post menopause" to define the years after the LMP. At this time, women who are having sexual intercourse with men can stop using contraception. In menopause, women who were taking hormones during perimenopause should have treatment reevaluated. Peripherally-produced sex hormones, such as estrone and androstenedione, play a more prominent role.

Q. Why don't all women experience menopausal symptoms?

A. Estrogen, progesterone, and testosterone receptors are present in all tissues in various concentrations and ratios. Polymorphisms in receptors and enzymes such as aromatase result in varying patterns. In addition to genetics, factors such as fat mass, exercise, exposure to alcohol, cigarettes, and other drugs may affect the appearance and/or degree of symptoms.

Q. Why isn't follicle stimulating hormone (FSH) a good test for menopause?

A. FSH and inhibin B, a regulator of FSH secretion, are unreliable for predicting reproductive phase. More recently, anti-Mullerian hormone (AMH) is being used to predict ovarian follicular reserve, but its application is more suited for fertility evaluation as opposed to identifying stages of menopausal transition. The following Fig. 1.3 shows the STRAW method, which is the preferred tool for identifying reproductive stages in perimenopausal women, without relying on either FSH or estradiol levels in isolation.

Q. How do surgical menopause, medical menopause, early menopause, and natural menopause differ?

A. Surgical menopause following oophorectomy results in an abrupt reduction of estrogens and progesterone that may require high initial doses of hormone therapy.

- Women who have undergone hysterectomy but have intact ovaries may not be able to distinguish perimenopause from menopause since they will not have menstrual bleeding.
- Medical menopause is due to destruction of ovaries due to radiation, chemotherapy, or drugs that block estrogen activity, such as tamoxifen. It may result in abrupt or gradual emergence of menopausal symptoms.
- Early menopause is generally defined as menopause by age 40–45. Surgical menopause differs from natural menopausal transition in that estradiol and progesterone concentrations are abruptly reduced; in natural menopause, progesterone decreases

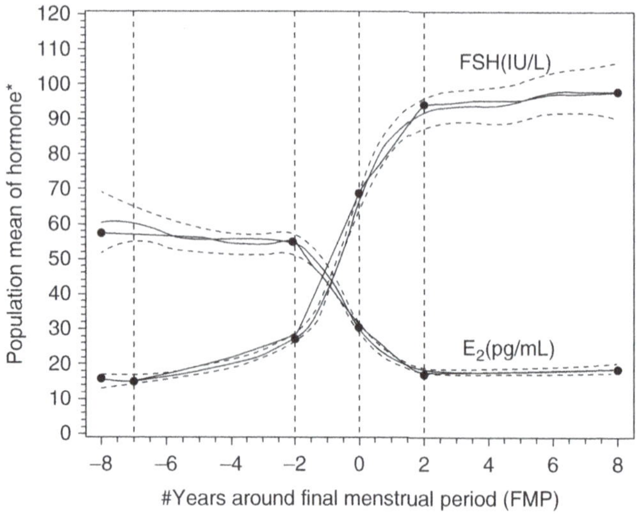

Fig. 1.3. STRAW: Identifying reproductive stages in perimenopausal women.

approximately around age 35 years, and estradiol levels spike erratically.

Q. What is the difference between the endogenous estrogens: estrone (E_1), estradiol (E_2), and estriol (E_3)?

A. The numbers refer to the quantity of hydroxyl side-chains. Estradiol has the most potent estrogen effect at the receptor level: 10 times more potent than estrone and 80 times more potent than estriol. The human ovarian granulosa cells produce 70–500 μg estradiol per day, depending upon the phase of the menstrual cycle. Estradiol is also produced in the brain, adrenal cortex, and vascular endothelium and, in pregnancy, the placenta. Estradiol is also formed by conversion from other sex hormones in the ovary, adrenal cortex, and adipocytes.

- Theca cells produce androstenedione which is converted to testosterone via aromatase (also in brain).
- Estrone, in turn, is converted to estradiol via 17-beta-hydroxysteroid dehydrogenase.

Typical serum concentrations of estradiol in premenopausal women range from:

- Follicular phase: 30–60 pg/mL
- Preovulatory: 100–400 pg/mL, mean 200

- Luteal phase: 20–150 pg/mL
- Menstruation: <50 pg/mL
- Perimenopausal: variable
- Postmenopausal: <35 pg/mL

Estrone (E_1) is manufactured by adipocytes. This is a medium-strength, proliferative estrogen. It is the primary estrogen produced after menopause; converted in body fat from androstenedione via aromatase. About 10% of estrogen in the body is in the form of estrone. The higher the number of adipocytes, the greater the serum concentrations of estrone.

Estradiol (E_2) is the source for Estrone and Estriol; progesterone causes it to be converted into the other two forms.

Estradiol is bound to sex hormone binding globulin (SHBG) and albumin. Free estradiol binds to the cytoplasmic estrogen receptor and then enters the nucleus where it exerts its effect via gene transcription.

Estriol (E_3) is the primary estrogen produced during pregnancy. It is non-proliferative. It is the weakest of the estrogens, with nearly 30% lower affinity for cells' estrogen receptor. Most estriol is converted from estrone in the liver. A small amount is converted from estradiol. An even smaller amount can be secreted directly from the ovaries.

After menopause, the main source of estrogen is estrone (E_1) from the adipocytes. This is especially true for patients who are obese. Estrogen is also stored in adipocytes, making prescription of HT to women who are obese a separate category, but also suggesting that women who are obese may have greater levels of endogenous estrogens that are relatively stable in perimenopause and may experience the stages of menopause differently from women who are not obese.

Q. Where are progesterone and testosterone produced?

A. Progesterone is produced by oocytes. In a premenopausal cycle, it is produced and dominant during days 14–28 of a menstrual cycle. When there is no ovulation, very little progesterone is produced. Progesterone production rises during puberty, cycles through the reproductive period, decreases fairly consistently during the perimenopausal years, and flattens in menopause.

Testosterone is found and produced in the ovaries, liver, skin, brain, and adrenals.

Q. What is the role of testosterone in HT?

A. Testosterone is prescribed for decreased libido in women. Transdermal testosterone patches have been shown to increase sexual activity modestly. Due to metabolic concerns, oral testosterone therapy is not recommended. It is reported that testosterone promotes a sense of well-being in young women's status post bilateral oophorectomy. Some clinicians aim for testosterone levels of 40–60 ng/mL.

Q. How do estrogens exert their influence?

A. Estrogen receptors exist in all tissues and estrogens have protean effects. Estrogens have both direct genomic and transcriptional activity. Among some of the known effects are:

- Neurogenic and neuroprotective effects
- Osteogenic effects
  - Antagonize parathyroid hormone
  - Suppress osteoclasts
- Gastrointestinal effects
  - Reduce bowel motility and increase absorption
- Metabolic effects
  - Improve insulin sensitivity in low doses but worsen in high doses
  - Increase the levels of SHBG
- Lipid effects
  - Exogenous oral estrogens increase HDL, apolipoprotein A, and triglycerides and decrease LDL, apolipoprotein B, and lipoprotein (a)
  - Alcohol ingestion increases estradiol levels
  - Estrogens given by transdermal routes of administration usually do not affect lipids
- Renal effects
  - Increases extracellular fluid and decreases intravascular space
  - Increases sodium and water retention
- Coagulability
  - In oral forms, estradiol increases coagulability and may unmask thrombophilias
- Immunologic
- Oral health
- Urogenital
  - Maintain structural integrity of uroepithelial and vaginal epithelial cell, including urethral sphincter tone
- Skin
  - Maintain structural integrity by increasing collagen formation
- Vascular
  - Upregulate nitric oxide synthetase and increased NO formation

Q. What is estrogen deficiency?

A. The widespread concept is that perimenopause is equivalent to estrogen "deficiency." In fact, estradiol serum and urine concentrations spike erratically during the perimenopause throughout the follicular phase and sometimes even during the luteal phase (a phenomenon described as luteal out-of-phase or LOOP events [Hale GE, Hughes CL, Burger HG, Robertson DM, Frazer IS. Atypical estradiol secretion and ovulation patterns caused by LOOP events underlying irregular ovulatory menstrual cycles in the menopausal transition. *Menopause* 16(1), 50–9, 2009]).

Despite normal, fluctuating, elevated, flat, or declining estradiol levels, menstrual cycles may be ovulatory or anovulatory. It is important to note that while estradiol may be in the normal range or increased during perimenopausal cycles, the level of progesterone is decreasing and the ratio of estradiol to progesterone is increasing. The physiologic changes that create typical symptoms may arise from:

- Elevated estradiol
- The rapid plummet of estradiol following the spike, and/or
- The steady reduction in progesterone, and/or
- The elevated estradiol to progesterone ratio, and/or
- Alterations in the estradiol to estrone ratio

Q. What is menopausal hormone therapy?

A. Menopausal Hormone Therapy (HT) refers to the prescription of either estrogen, progesterone, a combination of estrogen and progesterone, and occasionally testosterone, to treat menopausal symptoms. Current guidelines from medical associations are listed in Chap. 3.

Q. What are bioidentical hormones?

A. Bioidentical hormones are molecules that are the exact copy of endogenous sex hormones. Although commercial products have been on the market since the 1990s, the term "bioidentical hormones" is usually used to refer to only products prepared at compounding pharmacies. Compounded hormones have the advantage of being able to vary proportions of estradiol, estrone, estriol, progesterone, and testosterone. There are questions of efficacy of transdermal absorption and the quality control within individual pharmacies. Patients will frequently raise the question of "bioidentical hormones" with their physicians who may balk—they need to be reminded that "bioidentical" also refers to commercial products.

Estradiol has been available for years as both an oral formulation (Estrace®) and as a patch (Climara®, Vivelle®). Unlike oral estradiol, transdermal estradiol bypasses hepatic first-pass metabolism and presents intact to target tissues. Progesterone has been available since 1995 as oral micronized progesterone (Prometrium®) and, as an oral agent that undergoes first-pass metabolism, is converted to pregnenolone, among other compounds.

Q. How is estrogen loss related to other diseases of aging?

A. The questions of the relation of estrogen loss to diseases like osteoporosis, cardiovascular disease, cancer, and dementia/Alzheimers is tangled, with estrogen loss being but one of many factors that affect women's bodies as they age. These diseases have come to be seen as menopause-related (and before the 2002 WHI findings, were treated as such, with HT, before it was learned that HT exacerbated several of these conditions, and was only indicated for osteoporosis).

Q. Where are progesterone receptors located?

A. Progesterone affects these body systems. It helps stabilize blood sugar levels and appropriate cellular oxygen levels, as well as copper and zinc rations. It supports thyroid hormone and it supports thermogenesis.

- Central nervous system
- Breast and uterus
- Bone
- White blood cells
- Lungs
- Colon

Q. What is the difference between progesterone, progestogen, and progestin?

A. Progestogen is the term given for all progestin-like compounds, including endogenous progesterone and the exogenously administered progestins such as

- Medroxyprogesterone acetate (MPA)
- Norethindrone acetate (NETA)
- Norgestrel and levonorgesterol
- Drospirinone

Q. What is progesterone's effect in the body?

A. Among many of its known non-reproductive effects, progesterone affects

- Renal
  - Competitively antagonizes mineralocorticoids
  - Blunts effect of angiotensin II
- Neuronal
  - GABA receptor agonist
- Respiratory
  - Increases ventilator response to CO_2

Some progesterone deficiency symptoms include:

- Fluid retention
- Irritability
- Insomnia
- Infertility and pregnancy loss
- Menorrhagia
- Exacerbation of premenstrual syndrome symptoms

Q. What is the liver's role in the metabolism of estrogen and HT?

A. Liver metabolism has a crucially important effect on clinical prescription regarding routes of administration, especially in the last decade since 2002. All drugs eventually must pass through the liver so they can be filtered from the blood and metabolized into a form that can be eliminated via urine or bile. Oral estrogen/HT is absorbed directly into the liver, for circulation through the bloodstream. The liver breaks down large portions of the hormone before they can circulate through the body. The hormones then tend to be less effective. The also produce extra stress on the liver. Stress on the liver can cause elevated blood pressure and venusthromboembolism, nausea, headaches, and possibly weight gain and retention of fluids. This is one of the reasons for switching to transdermal HT, because it avoids first-pass liver metabolism.

Bibliography

1. Broer SL, Eijkemans JC, Scheffer GJ, et al. Anti-müllerian hormone predicts menopause: a long-term follow-up study in normoovulatory women. J Clin Endocrinol Metab. 2011;96(8):2532–9.
2. Crawford S, Santoro N, Laughlin GA, et al. Circulating dehydroepiandrosterone sulfate concentrations during the menopausal transition. J Clin Endocrinol Metab. 2009;94(8):2945–51.

3. Do Choi S, Steinberg EM, Hyeog Lee H, Naftolin F. The timing hypothesis remains a valid explanation of differential cardioprotective effects of menopausal hormone treatment [review article]. Menopause. 2011;18(2):230–6.
4. Freeman EW, Sammel MD, Lin H, Gracia CR. Anti-mullerian hormone as a predictor of time to menopause in late reproductive age women. J Clin Endocrinol Metab. 2012;97(5):1673–80.
5. Freeman WE, Sherif K. Prevalence of hot flushes and night sweats around the world: a systematic review. Climacteric. 2007;10:197–214.
6. Gast G-C M, Grobbee DE, Pop VJM, et al. Menopausal complaints are associated with cardiovascular risk factors. Hypertension. 2008;51(6):1492–8.
7. Gavin KM, Seals DR, Silver AE, Moreau KL. Vascular endothelial estrogen receptor alpha is modulated by estrogen status and related to endothelial function and eNOS in healthy women. J Clin Endocrinol Metab. 2009;94(9):3513–20.
8. Harlow SD, Gass M, Hall JE, et al. Executive summary of the Stages of Reproductive Aging Workshop + 10: addressing the unfinished agenda of staging reproductive aging. J Clin Endocrinol Metab. 2012;97(4):1159–68.
9. Harlow SD, Gass M, Hall JE, et al. Executive summary of the Stages of Reproductive Aging Workshop + 10: addressing the unfinished agenda of staging reproductive aging. Menopause. 2012;19(4):387–95.
10. Hunter MS, Gentry-Maharaj A, Ryan A, et al. Prevalence, frequency and problem rating of hot flushes persist in older postmenopausal women: impact of age, body mass index, hysterectomy, hormone therapy use, lifestyle and mood in a cross-sectional cohort study of 10 418 British women aged 54–65. BJOG. 2012;119(1):40–50.
11. Kok HS, van Asselt KM, van der Schouw YT, et al. Heart disease risk determines menopausal age rather than the reverse. J Am Coll Cardiol. 2006;47(10): 1976–83.
12. Konhilas JP, Leinwand LA. The effects of biological sex and diet on the development of heart failure. Circulation. 2007;116:2747–59.
13. Livingstone C, Collison M. Sex steroids and insulin resistance [review]. Clin Sci. 2002;102:151–66.
14. National Osteoporosis Foundation. 8 Common myths about osteoporosis. Washington, DC: National Osteoporosis Foundation; 2002.
15. Niland P, Lyons AC. Uncertainty in medicine: meanings of menopause and hormone replacement therapy in medical textbooks. Soc Sci Med. 2011;73:1238–45.
16. Notelovitz M. The clinical practice impact of the Women's Health Initiative: political vs biological correctness [guest editorial]. Maturitas. 2003;44:3–9.
17. Notelovitz M. The biological rationale for estrogen therapy. Presented at 25 April 2003, Adult Women's Health & Medicine meeting, Boca Raton, FL and Washington, DC.
18. O'Connor KA, Ferrell R, Brindle E, et al. Progesterone and ovulation across stages of the transition to menopause. Menopause. 2009;16(6):1178–87.
19. Phillips LS, Langer RD. Postmenopausal hormone therapy: critical reappraisal and a unified hypothesis. Fertil Steril. 2005;83(3):558–66.
20. Prior JC, Hitchcock CL. The endocrinology of perimenopause: need for a paradigm shift. Front Biosci. 2011;S3:474–86.

21. Rybaczyk LA, Bashaw MJ, Pathak DR, et al. An overlooked connection: serotonergic mediation of estrogen-related physiology and pathology. BMC Womens Health. 2005;5:12.
22. Salpeter SR, Walsh JME, Greyber E, Salpeter EE. Coronary heart disease events associated with hormone therapy in younger and older women: a meta-analysis [brief report]. J Gen Intern Med. 2006;12:363–6.
23. Santoro N, Crawford SL, Lasley WL. Factors related to declining luteal function in women during the menopausal transition. J Clin Endocrinol Metab. 2008;93(5): 1711–21.
24. Saraç F, Saydam G, Sahin F, et al. Effects of hormone therapy replacement on insulin resistance and platelet function tests. Med Princ Pract. 2009;18:43–7.
25. Sherif K. The effects of hormone replacement therapy and oral contraceptive pills on blood pressure. Prog Cardiovasc Nurs 2000;15(1):21–23,28.
26. Sherwin BB, Henry JF. Brain aging modulates the neuroprotective effects of estrogen on selective aspects of cognition in women: a critical review. Front Neuroendocrinol. 2008;29:88–113.
27. Szmuilowicz ED, Adler GK, Ricchiuti V, et al. Relationships between endogenous sex hormone concentrations and vascular function in postmenopausal women [brief report]. J Clin Endocrinol Metab. 2007;92(12):4738–41.
28. Erel T, Guralp O. Epilepsy and menopause. Arch Gynecol Obstet. 2011;284(3):749–55.
29. Taylor HS, Manson JE. Update in hormone therapy use in menopause. J Clin Endocrinol Metab. 2011;96(2):255–64.
30. Tepper PG, Randolph Jr JF, McConnell DS, et al. Trajectory clustering of estradiol and follicle-stimulating hormone during the menopausal transition among women in the Study of Women's Health across the nation (SWAN). Endocrine Res. 2012;97(8): 2872–80.
31. Thurston RC, Santoro N, Matthews KA. Adiposity and hot flashes in midlife women: a modifying role of age. J Clin Endocrinol Metab. 2011;96(10):E1588–95.
32. van de Weijer PHM. Risks of hormone therapy in the 50–59 year age group. Maturitas. 2008;60:59–64.
33. Wildman RP, Tepper PG, Crawford S, et al. Do changes in sex steroid hormones precede or follow increases in body weight during the menopause transition? Results from The Study of Women's Health Across the Nation. J Clin Endocrinol Metab. 2012;97(9):E1695–704.
34. Women's Health Initiative Investigators Writing Group. Risks and benefits of estrogen plus progestin in healthy postmenopausal women: principal results from the Women's Health Initiative randomized controlled trial. JAMA. 2002;288(3):321–33.
35. Xing D, Nozell S, Chen Y-F, et al. Estrogen and mechanisms of vascular protection. Arterioscler Thromb Vasc Biol. 2009;29:289–95.
36. Yamamoto H, Kitawaki J, Kikuchi N, et al. Effects of estrogens on cholinergic neurons in the rat basal nucleus. J Steroid Biochem Mol Biol. 2007;107:70–9.
37. Yang X-P, Reckelhoff JF. Estrogen, hormonal replacement therapy and cardiovascular disease. Curr Opin Nephrol Hypertens. 2011;20:133–8.
38. Zengin K, Tokac M, Akif Duzenli M, et al. Influence of menstrual cycle on cardiac performance. Maturitas. 2007;58:70–4.

2. Principles of Practice

Keywords Menopause • Transdermal estrogen • Hormone therapy prescription • Hormone therapy routes of administration

For decades, menopausal-range women have been treated as a homogenous subgroup, with HT seen as a one-size-fits-all prescription. Hormone therapy can no longer be expected to be the automatic prescription and "cure" for female aging that clinicians only a few years ago desired it to be. Today, HT and menopause management demand a focus on managing individual symptoms, paying close attention to what the patient reports, understanding the science, and helping patients demystify the many confusing popular reports they may have heard about menopause and about hormone therapies. The menopausal-range years offer a window of therapeutic opportunity, in which clinicians can help women move from their years of reproductive potential, to the postmenopausal period, with concern for symptomatic relief and general good health.

Principle of practice: *Menopause is not a disease, and should not be regarded as a pathophysiologic process.* If a woman presents with symptoms, these are treatable as such. There's no need to suffer through hot flashes, night sweats, cognitive problems, sleep disturbance, vaginal dryness, urinary incontinence, and other results of fluctuating levels of sex steroids. Conversely, women of menopausal age who don't have severe symptoms and who are doing just fine don't need HT just because they're in perimenopause or menopause.

Principle of practice: *The term "hormone therapy" is in many ways a misnomer, as is its implication that all estrogens are interchangeable.* Broad generalizations about hormone actions, efficacy, and safety greatly simplify a complex and nuanced body of knowledge.

K. Sherif, *Hormone Therapy: A Clinical Handbook*,
DOI 10.1007/978-1-4614-6268-2_2,

"Hormone therapy" is used to encompass all:

- Families of hormones, including estrogens (estradiol, estrone, and estriol), progesterone, and progestins (such as medroxyprogesterone acetate) and testosterone
- Types of estrogens, ranging from conjugated equine estrogens and plant-derived esterified to bioidentical
- Types of progesterone and progestins, including, among others, medroxyprogesterone acetate, NETA, and oral micronized progesterone
- Routes of administration, including oral, transdermal, intravaginal, local topical and coming, injections subdermal pellets and soon, inhalations
- Dosing regimens, including daily and cyclic
- Broad statements about hormone safety and efficacy greatly simplify a complex and nuanced area

Priniciple of practice: *<u>The perimenopausal transition is not equivalent to estrogen deficiency but involves changes in other sex steroids including progesterone, testosterone, and their ratios.</u>* In some women, estradiol levels may be higher in perimenopausal cycles compared to their premenopausal cycles. It is essential that clinicians recognize that the symptoms arise from changes in sex hormones, not just deficiency. These changes include a steady decrease in progesterone production and an increase in the estradiol to progesterone ratio until the last cessation of cycles.

Principle of practice: *<u>Women experience the menopausal years as individuals, and require individualized medical care and hormone therapy.</u>* Women have varied perimenopausal symptoms that may occur as early as their late thirties and postmenopausal symptoms that can occur as late as their sixties. These require varied treatment. Even women of similar age respond differently to various formulations, dosing regimens, and routes of administration. Necessary for effective hormone therapy is a focus on treating individuals, not populations. Currently, there are few specific guidelines for prescribing hormones, and there are none that instruct how to individualize the care that perimenopausal and postmenopausal women receive. This handbook rectifies that knowledge gap with easy to access information about dosage, drugs, routes of administration, and decision-making based on symptoms. The one-time practice of a standardized and uniform approach to menopause treatment is outdated. Women experience symptoms differently and must be treated accordingly.

Below are additional principles of practice for perimenopause and postmenopausal management and HT prescription:

- HT should not be used to "treat" or prevent other disease associated with aging, including heart disease and cancer risk.
- HT should be used specifically to alleviate symptoms of perimenopause and menopause, including hot flushes and night sweats, cognitive "fuzziness", urogenital symptoms, and sleep disturbance.
- The well-publicized dangers of a prior generation of hormone replacement therapy in terms of raised risks of breast cancer and heart disease were based on the use of a specific formulation of oral conjugated equine estrogens and medroxyprogesterone acetate. Not only were the conclusions based upon two popular regimens, but the negative findings of increased incidence of breast cancer and coronary artery disease were not detected in women who started hormones in their 40s and 50s. The new favored prescription practice is transdermal application, either through patch, cream, or gel.
- Women understandably may be very skeptical about using hormones given the amount of controversial and often conflicting media attention accorded to the WHI findings. Women may require a great deal of explanation about risks and benefits. The important principle is to work in partnership with patients, giving them enough information so that they can make informed decisions about this controversial area.
- Many clinicians have been reluctant to prescribe hormones due to a pronounced lack of coverage given to the WHI findings of safety and benefits in younger women.
- Women in the menopausal range have a huge amount of information at their fingertips due to the popularity of books by Dr. Susan Love and celebrity Suzanne Somers about aging and about designer bioidentical hormones. The medical information in Somers's books is relatively sound, even if in our opinion and in most cases the designer estrogen phenomenon is not more effective than the new HT practice. The most important thing we practitioners need to do and know is to be respectful of the information about bioidentical hormones that our female patients are bringing into our offices, and work with them from that basis as we provide sound medical guidance for prescribing and monitoring HT use.

Bibliography

1. Bechlioulis A, Naka KK, Kalantaridou SN, et al. Increased vascular inflammation in early menopausal women is associated with hot flush severity. J Clin Endocrinol Metab. 2012;97(5):E760–4.
2. Collins P, Rosano G, Casey C, et al. Management of cardiovascular risk in the peri-menopausal woman: a consensus statement of European cardiologists and gynaecologists. Eur Heart J. 2007;28:2028–40.
3. Cumming GP, Currie HD, Panay N, et al. Stopping hormone replacement therapy: were women ill advised? Menopause Int. 2011;17:82–7.
4. Hisamoto K, Bender JR. Vascular cell signaling by membrane estrogen receptors. Steroids. 2005;70:382–7.
5. Ichikawa A, Sumino H, Ogawa T, et al. Effects of long-term transdermal hormone replacement therapy on the renin-angiotensin-aldosterone system, plasma bradykinin levels and blood pressure in normotensive postmenopausal women. Geriatr Gerontol Int. 2008;8:259–64.
6. Kuhl H. Mechanisms of sex steroids: future developments. Maturitas. 2004;47: 285–91.
7. Maki PM, Dennerstein L, Clark M. Perimenopausal use of hormone therapy is associated with enhanced memory and hippocampal function later in life. Brain Res. 2011;1379:232–43.
8. Mong JA, Baker FC, Mahoney MM, et al. Sleep, rhythms, and the endocrine brain: influence of sex and gonadal hormones. J Neurosci. 2011;31(45):16107–16.
9. Morgan ML, Cook IA, Rapkin AJ, Leuchter AF. Neurophysiologic changes during estrogen augmentation in perimenopausal depression. Maturitas. 2007;56:54–60.
10. Ostberg JE, Storry C, Donald AE, et al. A dose–response study of hormone replacement in young hypogonadal women: effects on intima media thickness and metabolism. Clin Endocrinol. 2007;66:557–64.
11. Pluchino N, Bucci F, Cela V, et al. Menopause and mental well-being: timing of symptoms and timing of hormone treatment. Womens Health (Lond Engl). 2011;7(1): 71–80.
12. Practice Committee of the American Society for Reproductive Medicine. Estrogen and progestogen therapy in postmenopausal women. Fertil Steril. 2008;90 suppl 3: S88–102.
13. Archer DF. Progestogens: effects on clinical and biochemical parameters in postmenopausal women. Menopause. 2005;12(5):484–7.
14. Prossnitz ER, Oprea TI, Sklar LA, Arterburn JB. The ins and outs of GPR30: a transmembrane estrogen receptor. J Steroid Biochem Mol Biol. 2008;109(3–5): 350–3.

3. Medical Association Guidelines, Post-2002/Women's Health Initiative Findings

Keywords Hormone therapy • FDA • North American Menopause Society • International Menopause Society • American Association of Clinical Endocrinology

The findings of the NIH's Women's Health Initiative Study in 2002 changed forever the way that HT had been understood to work and the wide range of benefits it was thought to have provided. In the decade since, researchers and practitioners have come to understand safer ways to prescribe estrogen and estrogen plus progesterone replacement therapy so that women seeking relief from menopause symptoms can access a safe hormone therapy that relieves symptoms without suffering from unwanted and dangerous side effects.

The WHI findings raised immediate concerns about oral HT risk. This prompted medical and scientific associations and regulatory agencies to revise their HT recommendations and formulations of therapeutic value versus risk for HT. Side effects and risks are now better understood and can be factored into medical decision-making.

At times these guidelines can be confusing and even contradictory, and they often are not specific enough for prescription use. They are reported here, as they provide the professional context for the new transdermal hormone replacement therapy. Please note the third set of guidelines, too, from the European-based International Menopause Society.

K. Sherif, *Hormone Therapy: A Clinical Handbook*,
DOI 10.1007/978-1-4614-6268-2_3,

FDA Approvals and Contraindications

FDA Approvals for HT

Approval 1	The treatment of moderate to severe vasomotor symptoms of menopause, including hot flushes and night sweats. The FDA has not changed this approval even after the WHI studies that questioned the safety levels of postmenopausal women. The most effective therapy for these symptoms is estrogen replacement
Approval 2	The treatment of moderate to severe symptoms of vaginal and vulvar atrophy related to menopause, including dryness, itching, and burning. Topical vaginal regimens should be prescribed when the major symptom is vaginal and vulvar
Approval 3	HT may be prescribed for osteoporosis related to post-menopause, but when this is the sole reason for its prescription, non-estrogen treatments should be considered first. Only when the risk of osteoporosis is severe enough to outweigh the risks of long-term use of estrogen and estrogen plus progesterone use should HT be prescribed for the prevention of osteoporosis

FDA Contraindications for HT

1. Breast cancer: current, history, or suspected high risk
2. Suspected or known malignant conditions that are estrogen-sensitive
3. Undiagnosed genital bleeding
4. Untreated endometrial hyperplasia
5. Previous idiopathic or current venous thromboembolism, including deep vein thrombosis, pulmonary embolism
6. Active or recent arterial thromboembolic disease, including angina, myocardial infarction
7. Untreated hypertension
8. Acute liver disease
9. Known hypersensitivity to the active substances of HT or any of the excipients
10. Porphyria cutanea tarda (absolute contraindication)

Source: Approvals and Contraindications taken from 2011 AACE Medical Guidelines for Clinical Practice for the Diagnosis and Treatment of Menopause https://www.aace.com/sites/default/files/menopause.pdf

The North American Menopause Society

The North American Menopause Society (NAMS) Guidelines

(Note: NAMS uses abbreviations HT for Hormone Therapy, ET for Estrogen Therapy, EPT for Estrogen and Progesterone Therapy)

1. Individualization is of key importance in the decision to use HT and should incorporate the woman's health and quality of life priorities as well as her personal risk factors, such as risk of venous thrombosis, CHD, stroke, and breast cancer
2. The recommendation for duration of therapy differs for EPT and ET. For EPT, duration is limited by the increased risk of breast cancer and breast cancer mortality associated with 3–5 years of use; for ET, a more favorable benefit- risk profile was observed during a mean of 7 years of use and 4 years of follow-up, a finding that allows more flexibility in duration of use
3. ET is the most effective treatment of symptoms of vulvar and vaginal atrophy; low-dose, local vaginal ET is advised when only vaginal symptoms are present
4. Women with premature or early menopause who are otherwise appropriate candidates for HT can use HT at least until the median age of natural menopause (age 51 years). Longer duration of treatment can be considered if needed for symptom management
5. Although ET did not increase breast cancer risk in the WHI, there is a lack of safety data supporting the use of ET in breast cancer survivors, and one RCT reported a higher increase in breast cancer recurrence rates
6. Both transdermal and low-dose oral estrogen have been associated with lower risks of VTE and stroke than standard doses of oral estrogen, but RCT evidence is not yet available

Source: The 2012 Hormone Therapy Position Statement of the North American Menopause Society http://www.menopause.org/psht12.pdf NAMS POSITION STATEMENT Menopause, Vol. 19, No. 3.

International Menopause Society: Recommendations on Postmenopausal Hormonal Therapy and Preventative Strategies for Midlife Health

(Adapted from: Updated IMS recommendations on postmenopausal hormone therapy and preventive strategies for midlife health. International Menopause Society *Climacteric* 2011;14:302–20)

Introduction

- The 2011 revision of the IMS Recommendations is published when the atmosphere around the issue of postmenopausal HRT is much more rational.
- This document has been produced by a small Writing Group of experts, but is the considered view of the IMS on the principles of HRT in the peri- and postmenopausal periods.
- The term HRT will be used to cover therapies including estrogens, progestogens, combined therapies, androgens, and tibolone.
- The IMS is aware of the geographical variations related to different priorities of medical care, different prevalence of diseases, and country-specific attitudes of the public, the medical community, and the health authorities toward menopause management, different availability and licensing of products, all of which may impact on HRT.
- These Recommendations therefore give a global and simple overview on issues related to the various aspects of hormone treatment, which can be easily adapted and modified according to local needs.

Governing Principles

- Consideration of HRT should be part of an overall strategy including lifestyle recommendations regarding diet, exercise, smoking cessation, and safe levels of alcohol consumption for maintaining the health of peri- and postmenopausal women.
- HRT should not be recommended without a clear indication for its use, i.e., significant symptoms or physical effects of estrogen deficiency.
- Postmenopausal HRT is not a single regimen given to a standard woman.

- HRT must be individualized and tailored according to symptoms and the need for prevention, as well as personal and family history, results of relevant investigations, the woman's preferences and expectations.

Early Menopause

- Women experiencing a spontaneous or iatrogenic menopause before the age of 45 years and particularly before 40 years are at higher risk for cardiovascular disease and osteoporosis and may be at increased risk of affective disorders and dementia. Use of HRT may reduce these risks but the evidence for this is limited. HRT may reduce symptoms and preserve bone density and is advised at least until the average age of menopause.

Class Effect

- HRT includes a wide range of hormonal products and routes of administration, with potentially different risks and benefits. Thus, the term "class effect" is confusing and inappropriate. However, evidence regarding differences in risks and benefits between different products is limited.

Duration of Therapy

- There are no reasons to place mandatory limitations on the duration of HRT. Whether or not to continue therapy should be decided at the discretion of the well-informed woman and her health professional, dependent upon the specific goals and an objective estimation of ongoing benefits and risks.
- Women can have the option of HRT for as long as they derive symptomatic benefit and are aware of the risks for their regimen and personal circumstances. They can try without HRT every few years, but menopausal symptoms in some women can last for many years and should be treated with the lowest effective dose.

Dosage

- Dosage should be titrated to the lowest effective dose. Lower doses of HRT than have been used previously may reduce symptoms sufficiently and maintain quality of life for many women. Long-term data on lower doses regarding fracture or cancer risks and cardiovascular implications are still lacking.

The Age Factor

- The safety of HRT largely depends on age.
- The risks and benefits of HRT differ for women during the menopause transition compared to those for older women.

Safety Considerations

- Healthy women younger than 60 years should not be unduly concerned about the safety profile of HRT. New data and re-analyses of older studies by women's age show that, for most women, the potential benefits of HRT given for a clear indication are many and the risks are few when initiated within a few years of menopause.

Counseling

- Women taking HRT should have at least an annual consultation to include a physical examination, update of medical and family history, relevant laboratory and imaging investigations, a discussion on lifestyle, and strategies to prevent or reduce chronic disease. There is currently no indication for increased mammographic or cervical smear screening.
- Counseling should convey the benefits and risks of HRT in clear and comprehensible terms, e.g., as absolute numbers rather than, or in addition to, percentage changes from baseline expressed as a relative risk. This allows a woman and her physician to make a well-informed decision about HRT. Written information about risks and benefits as well as decision aids may be useful.

Progestogens, Reasons for Use

- In general, progestogen should be added to systemic estrogen for all women with a uterus to prevent endometrial hyperplasia and cancer.
- Low-dose vaginal estrogens, administered for the relief of urogenital atrophy, are systemically absorbed, but not at levels that stimulate the endometrium, and so concurrent progestogen is not required.

Progestogens, Safety Considerations

- The Women's Health Initiative (WHI) and other studies strongly suggest that it is the progestogen component of HRT that is more significant in any increase in breast cancer risk rather than the estrogen. Thus, it seems prudent to minimize progestogen use where safely possible and, in the near future, progestogens may be replaced by selective estrogen receptor modulators (SERMs) that do not adversely affect the breast, but also inhibit endometrial proliferation.

Progestogens, Other Effects

- Natural progesterone and some progestogens have specific beneficial effects that could justify their use besides the expected actions on the endometrium, e.g., the well-documented blood pressure-lowering effect of drospirenone.
- Progestogens may not be alike in regard to potential adverse metabolic effects or associated breast cancer risk when combined with long-term estrogen therapy.

Androgen Therapy

- Androgen replacement should be reserved for women with clinical signs and symptoms of androgen insufficiency.
- Androgen replacement often has significant beneficial effects in women with bilateral oophorectomy or adrenal failure, particularly on health-related quality of life and sexual function.

Benefits of HRT: General

- HRT remains the most effective therapy for vasomotor symptoms and urogenital atrophy.
- Other menopause-related complaints, such as joint and muscle pains, mood swings, sleep disturbances, and sexual dysfunction (including reduced libido), may improve during HRT.

Benefits of HRT: Urogenital Symptoms

- Symptoms such as vaginal dryness, soreness, dyspareunia, urinary frequency, nocturia, and urgency are extremely common in postmenopausal women. Incontinence in women increases in prevalence with age.
- Systemic HRT can correct estrogen deficiency changes in the urogenital tract and maintain vaginal health.
- All local estrogen preparations are effective and patient preference will usually determine the treatment used.

- Urogenital symptoms respond well to estrogens.
- Long-term treatment is often required as symptoms can recur on cessation of therapy.
- Use of systemic HRT does not seem to prevent urinary incontinence and is not preferable to low-dose local estrogens in the management of urogenital atrophy or recurrent lower urinary tract infections.

Benefits of HRT: Postmenopausal Osteoporosis

- HRT is effective in preventing bone loss associated with the menopause and decreases the incidence of all osteoporosis-related fractures, including vertebral and hip fractures, even in women not at high risk of fracture.
- Based on evidence of effectiveness, cost and safety, HRT can be considered as one of the first-line therapies for the prevention and treatment of osteoporosis in postmenopausal women, younger than 60 years, with an increased risk of fracture.
- The initiation of HRT for the sole purpose of the prevention of fractures after the age 60 years is not recommended.
- Continuation of HRT after the age of 60 years for the sole purpose of the prevention of fractures should take into account the possible long-term effects of the specific dose and method of administration of HRT, compared to other proven nonhormonal therapies.
- The protective effect of HRT on bone mineral density declines after cessation of therapy at an unpredictable rate, although some degree of fracture protection may remain after cessation of HRT.
- If the patient is still considered at risk for fracture after cessation of HRT, additional therapy with proven bone-sparing medication should be given.
- Evidence of the fracture-protective effect of HRT is limited to standard dosages of conjugated equine estrogen (CEE) and medroxyprogesterone acetate (MPA), given by the oral route. Evidence for protection against loss of bone mineral density is available for lower than standard doses in oral (CEE and 17β-estradiol) and transdermal (17β-estradiol) administration.
- Tibolone, a synthetic molecule that has affinity for the estrogen, progesterone, and androgen receptors, has proven efficacy against vertebral and non-vertebral fractures.

- The SERMs, raloxifene, lasofoxifene, and bazedoxifene, reduce the risk of vertebral fracture in postmenopausal women with or without prevalent vertebral fractures.
- A combination of bazedoxifene and CEE has been shown to preserve bone mineral density.

Benefits of HRT: Connective Tissues

- Intervertebral discs become thinner after the menopause and this may be prevented by estrogen therapy.
- After the menopause, there is loss of connective tissue in the dermis of the skin which in some cases is reversed with estrogen therapy.
- Timely initiation of estrogen treatment can effectively prevent cartilage loss accompanying the menopause, involving both direct and indirect mechanisms.

Benefits of HRT: Colorectal Cancer

- In the WHI randomized, controlled trial of estrogen and progestogen therapy, colorectal cancer risk was reduced (relative risk 0.56). This effect was predominantly for local disease and, where spread had occurred, there was more node involvement and a more advanced stage at diagnosis among users of HRT.
- Results from the WHI randomized trial of estrogen-only therapy showed no effect of estrogen-only therapy on risk of colorectal cancer.
- The majority of observational studies show a reduced risk of colorectal cancer among users of oral HRT.
- Three meta-analyses have reported a reduced risk of colorectal cancer with HRT use with benefit persisting for 4 years after cessation of therapy.
- There are no data for an effect of non-oral HRT on risk of colorectal cancer.

Benefits of HRT: Cardiovascular Disease

- Menopause may be considered a risk factor for coronary artery disease in women due to the potential effects of ovarian failure on cardiovascular function, blood pressure, and various metabolic parameters (glucose tolerance, lipid profile).

- Arterial hypertension, high triglyceride level, and diabetes are more important cardiovascular risk factors in women than in men.
- Once they develop an infarct, the prognosis in women is significantly worse than that in men.
- HRT has the potential for improving the cardiovascular risk profile through its beneficial effects on vascular function, cholesterol levels, glucose metabolism, and blood pressure.
- HRT reduces the risk of diabetes and, through improving insulin action in women with insulin resistance, it has positive effects on other related risk factors for cardiovascular disease such as the metabolic syndrome.
- There is evidence that estrogen therapy may be cardioprotective if started around the time of menopause and continued long term (often referred to as the "window of opportunity" concept).
- In women less than 60 years old, recently menopausal and without evidence of cardiovascular disease, the initiation of HRT does not cause early harm and may reduce morbidity and mortality from coronary heart disease.
- Continuation of HRT beyond the age of 60 years should be decided as a part of the overall risk–benefit analysis.
- Initiation of HRT in elderly women or those who are more than 10 years postmenopause may be associated with increased risk for coronary events, mainly in the first 2 years of use.
- It is not recommended to initiate HRT beyond the age of 60 years solely for the purpose of primary prevention of coronary artery disease.
- It is well accepted that initiation of HRT is not appropriate in the routine treatment of older women with coronary disease.

Benefits of HRT: Dementia

- Observational evidence implies that HRT used by younger women around the time of menopause is associated with lower risk of Alzheimer's disease.
- Limited clinical trial evidence indicates that HRT increases all-cause dementia risk when initiated in the late postmenopause. For women aged 65–79 years, the excess risk of dementia attributed to hormone use is about 1.2 per 1,000 person-years for estrogen therapy and 2.3 per 1,000 person-years for estrogen plus progestogen therapy.

Benefits of HRT: Cognition

- Limited evidence from short-term clinical trials in midlife women suggests that HRT has no substantial cognitive effect after natural menopause.
- For older women without cognitive impairment, there is convincing clinical trial evidence that HRT started in the late postmenopause has no substantial impact on cognitive abilities.
- For surgically menopausal women, limited evidence from small clinical trials suggests that estrogen therapy could be of short-term cognitive benefit when initiated at the time of oophorectomy.

Adverse Effects: Stroke

- The risk of stroke is correlated with age, but stroke is a rare event before age 60.
- HRT may further increase that risk, becoming significant after the age of 60.
- Low-dose transdermal preparations are not associated with increased risk for stroke.
- Safety data from studies of low-dose and ultra-low-dose regimens of estrogen and progestogen are encouraging, with fewer adverse events, but data from large prospective trials are awaited.

Adverse Effects: Venous Thromboembolism

- The HRT-related risk for serious venous thromboembolic events increases with age (although minimal in low-risk women until age 60) and is also positively associated with obesity and thrombophilia.
- Transdermal estrogen may avert the risk associated with oral HRT by avoiding first-pass hepatic metabolism.
- The impact on the risk of a thromboembolic event may also be affected by the type of progestogen.

Adverse Effects: Breast Cancer

- The incidence of breast cancer varies in different countries. Therefore, currently available data may not be applicable everywhere. The degree of association between breast cancer and postmenopausal HRT remains controversial.

- Women should be reassured that the possible increased risks of breast cancer associated with HRT are small (an incidence of <1.0 per 1,000 women per year of use), and less than the increased risks associated with common lifestyle factors such as obesity and alcohol consumption.
- Randomized controlled data from the WHI study demonstrated no increased risk in first-time users of combined HRT during the 5–7 years since initiation of treatment.
- Data from the WHI and the Nurses' Health Study suggest that long-term, estrogen-only administration for 7 and 15 years, respectively, does not increase the risk of breast cancer in North American women.
- Recent European observational studies suggest that the risk may increase after 5 years.
- There are insufficient data to evaluate the possible differences in the incidence of breast cancer using different types, doses and routes of estrogen, natural progesterone, and progestogens and androgen administration.
- Nevertheless, large European observational studies suggest that a difference in risk between estrogen-only and combined estrogen–progestogen therapy is seen with some categories of progestogens but not with natural progesterone derivatives.
- The concomitant dramatic decrease in HRT use and the immediate reduction in breast cancer incidence post-WHI in some studies were presented as further proof of the carcinogenic effect of estrogen.
- However, recent data indicate an increase in breast cancer incidence despite stabilization in the number of HRT users, suggesting that HRT may be a promoter of an existing breast tumor rather than an initiator of cancer.

Adverse Effects: Mammography

- Baseline mammographic density correlates with breast cancer risk. This does not necessarily apply to the increase in mammographic density induced by HRT.
- The combined estrogen–progestogen therapy-related increase in mammographic density may impede the diagnostic interpretation of mammograms.

Adverse Effects: Endometrium

- Unopposed estrogen administration induces a dose-related stimulation of the endometrium. Women with a uterus should have progestogen supplementation to counteract this effect.
- Continuous combined estrogen–progestogen regimens are associated with a lower incidence of endometrial hyperplasia and cancer than occurs in the normal population.
- Long-cycle regimens and long-term use of monthly sequential regimens do not provide optimal endometrial protection.
- Regimens containing low-/ultra-low-dose estrogen and progestogen cause less endometrial stimulation and less bleeding.
- Direct delivery of progestogen to the endometrial cavity from the vagina or by an intrauterine system does provide endometrial protection and may cause less systemic progestogenic effects than other routes of administration.
- Data from randomized controlled trials on the effect of tibolone on the endometrium suggest a similar effect to continuous combined regimens.
- Tamoxifen has an estrogenic effect on the endometrium, whereas raloxifene and other modern SERMs have no apparent effect.

Adverse Effects: Ovarian Cancer

- Long-term estrogen-only therapy may be associated with a small attributable risk of ovarian cancer of 0.7 per 1,000 women per 5 years of use, while either a significantly smaller, or no, increased risk is seen with combined estrogen plus progestogen therapy.
- Long-term estrogen-only therapy may be associated with a small attributable risk of ovarian cancer of 0.7 per 1,000 women per 5 years of use, while either a significantly smaller, or no, increased risk is seen with combined estrogen plus progestogen therapy.

Nonhormonal Therapies: Vasomotor Symptoms

- Selective serotonin reuptake inhibitors (SSRI), selective noradrenaline reuptake inhibitors (SNRI), and gabapentin are effective in reducing vasomotor symptoms in short-term studies. Their long-term safety needs further evaluation.
- High-quality studies to date have not supported the efficacy of complementary or over-the-counter therapies in reducing severity or frequency of hot flushes or night sweats.

- Black cohosh and soy products are not superior to placebo in the treatment of hot flushes.

Alternative Treatments

- The efficacy and safety of complementary alternative medicines have not been demonstrated and further studies are required.
- There are no medical or scientific reasons to recommend unregistered "bioidentical hormones." The measurement of hormone levels in the saliva is not clinically useful. These "customized" hormonal preparations have not been adequately tested in studies and their purity and risks are unknown.

AACE/American Association of Clinical Endocrinology

AACE Guidelines for MRT

(Note: The AACE refers to HT as MRT, Menopause Replacement Therapy)

Number	Recommendation	Grade
1	MHT may be appropriate for the relief of severe menopausal symptoms in selected postmenopausal women, on the basis of an individually determined benefit vs. risk profile	Grade A; BEL 1
2	MHT may be prescribed during the perimenopause and early menopause for relief of menopausal symptoms and treatment of vulvovaginal atrophy	Grade A; BEL 1
3	The use of the transdermal route of estrogen administration should be considered in order to avoid the hepatic "first-pass effect," which may theoretically reduce the risk of thromboembolic disease	Grade B; BEL 3
4	The use of transvaginal estrogen may be considered to provide topical effects with less systemic absorption	Grade B; BEL 3
5	The dose of MHT may be reduced with advancing age	Grade C; BEL 3
6	Because of the increased risk of endometrial cancer, unopposed estrogen should not be used in women with an intact uterus	Grade D; BEL 1

(continued)

Number	Recommendation	Grade
7	Progestational agents should be used for a minimum of 10–14 days per month in women treated with estrogen who have an intact uterus	Grade A; BEL 1
8	Long-cycle therapy with use of a progestagen for 14 days every 3 months may be considered, in an effort to reduce breast exposure to progestagens, despite lack of definitive assessment of efficacy	Grade B; BEL 2
9	Amenorrhea may be achieved by using a low dose of a progestagen administered continuously (daily) in conjunction with estrogen. Because recent studies suggest adverse breast outcomes with continuous progesterone exposure, this form of therapy is not recommended	Grade D; BEL 2
10	MHT should be used in the lowest dose and for the shortest period necessary to control menopausal symptoms	Grade A; BEL 1
11	Therapeutic trials of nonhormonal prescription medications, including clonidine, antidepressants (selective serotonin reuptake inhibitors), and gabapentin, may be considered for the relief of menopausal symptoms in women with no specific contraindications	Grade B; BEL 2
12	Over-the-counter supplements should be used with caution because they are not regulated by the US Food and Drug Administration (FDA) and have the potential for interactions with drugs and for causing harm	Grace C; BEL 2
13	Phytoestrogens, including soy-derived isoflavonoids, result in inconsistent relief of symptoms. Because these compounds may have estrogenic effects, women with a personal or strong family history of hormone- dependent cancers (breast, uterine, or ovarian), thromboembolic events, or cardiovascular events should not use soy-based therapies	Grade D; BEL 1
14	Custom compounded "bioidentical hormone therapy" is not recommended	Grade D; BEL 1
15	FDA-approved bioidentical hormone preparations may be considered, but evidence is lacking that they are safer or more effective than traditional forms of hormone therapy	Grade C; BEL 2

(continued)

Number	Recommendation	Grade
16	MHT should be used for the prevention and treatment of osteoporosis within the context of the overall benefit-versus-risk analysis of each patient. Data from multiple randomized controlled trials (RCTs) substantiate the efficacy of estrogens in preserving bone mass and, less consistently, preventing fractures, but nonhormonal therapeutic options for bone health exist	Grade A; BEL 1
17	Hormone therapy for the prevention or treatment (or both) of dementia is not recommended	Grade D; BEL 1
18	MHT should be prescribed to women in conjunction with a thorough discussion of the possible relationship of MHT to breast cancer. Current evidence suggests that E+P regimens are associated with a possible higher risk of breast cancer than is therapy with estrogen alone	Grade A; BEL 1
19	Concordant with current FDA warnings, we recommend that women who are at increased risk of thromboembolic disease should not take estrogen-containing therapy (although there is evidence that transdermal estradiol may not increase this risk; see subsequent material)	Grade D; BEL 1
20	Women should be advised that smoking increases the risk of cardiovascular and venous thromboembolic disease when taking estrogen, and aggressive smoking cessation programs should be advised	Grade A; BEL 1
21	MHT is not recommended for primary or secondary prevention of cardiovascular disease	Grade D; BEL 1
22	Lipid profiles, smoking history, and diabetes history as well as family history should be assessed to assist in the determination of individual cardiovascular risk	Grade A; BEL 1
23	Women should be advised that cerebrovascular accidents occur with increased frequency in patients taking estrogen alone or E+P combination therapies in an age-dependent manner	Grade A; BEL 1
24	Women should be advised that there may be an increase in ovarian epithelial tumors with the use of estrogen for more than 10 years	Grade B; BEL 2
25	Women may be advised that several studies including the Women's Health Initiative (WHI) have demonstrated a lower risk of colon cancer in women treated with E+P combination	Grade B; BEL 2

Source: Approvals and Contraindications taken from 2011 AACE Medical Guidelines for Clinical Practice for the Diagnosis and Treatment of Menopause https://www.aace.com/sites/default/files/menopause.pdf

Bibliography

1. ACOG Committee on Gynecologic Practice. Committee opinion number 322, November 2005. Compounded bioidentical hormones. Obstet Gynecol 2005;106(5 part 1): 1139–40.
2. North American Menopause Society. Position statement: Estrogen and progestogen use in postmenopausal women: 2010 position statement of The North American Menopause Society. Menopause. 2010;17(2):242–55.
3. Santen RJ, Allred DC, Ardoin SP, et al. Executive summary: postmenopausal hormone therapy: an Endocrine Society scientific statement. J Clin Endocrinol Metab. 2010;95 suppl 1:S1–66.
4. Sturdee DW, Pines A, International Menopause Society Writing Group, et al. Updated IMS recommendations on postmenopausal hormone therapy and preventive strategies for midlife health. Climacteric 2011;14:302–20.
5. Sturdee DW, Pines A, on behalf of the International Menopause Society Writing Group. Updated IMS recommendations on postmenopausal hormone therapy and preventive strategies for midlife health. Climacteric 2011;14:302–20.

4. Perimenopausal Symptoms: Hot Flushes and Night Sweats; Sleep Disturbances; Urogenital Discomfort; Sexual Libido Issues; Mood and Cognitive Changes

Keywords Hot flushes • Hot flashes • Menopause symptoms • Mood changes • Night sweats

Introduction

From a physiological standpoint estrogen and progesterone deficiency cause a variety of changes in the body, many of which are subtle and wouldn't be noticed by our patients. Here's what your patients will report as the troubling symptoms they associate with perimenopause and postmenopause.

Most Common Perimenopausal Symptoms that Women Report

Symptom	Comment
Menstrual	Irregular periods, shorter intervals, menorrhagia, worsening of PMS
Vasomotor	Hot flushes, night sweats, palpitations
Sleep	Decreased quality of sleep, daytime fatigue, longer latency to sleep, interrupted sleep
Mood	Depression, anxiety, emotional lability, recurrence of bipolar disorder
Cognitive	Decreased short term memory and concentration. "Fuzziness."

(continued)

K. Sherif, *Hormone Therapy: A Clinical Handbook*,
DOI 10.1007/978-1-4614-6268-2_4,

Symptom	Comment
Urogenital	Vaginal atrophy, urinary stress/incontinence, urinary frequency, recurrent cystitis, vaginal dryness, pruritus vulvae, dyspareunia
Sexual	Decreased libido, decrease in sexual sensation, diminished orgasm, delay in orgasm

Additional Symptoms that Women Report and Often Associate with Menopause and Postmenopause

There are additional perimenopausal and postmenopausal symptoms that are not primarily treated with hormone replacement therapy. These include:

Symptom	Comment
Alopecia	
Burning tongue and mouth	
Tinnitus	
Increase in allergy sensitivity	
Weight gain	Especially abdominal
Muscle and joint pain	
Vocal quality	
Aging skin	Changes in skin tone
General achiness	

These symptoms would rarely be sufficient to prescribe HT without the presence of the primary symptoms

Vasomotor Symptoms: Hot Flushes/Night Sweats

Vasomotor symptoms include hot flushes and sweats. Hot flushes are often described as an abrupt warm or hot sensation, often starting in the face and scalp and radiating downwards. Hot flushes are often followed by sweating. Hot flushes vary in frequency, intensity, and time of day. They may be very intense and uncomfortable and cause drenching sweats, or they may be mild. The frequency may vary from minutes to hours, or occur primarily at night. Nocturnal hot flushes may be accompanied by palpitations. In an individual, there may be changing patterns, in which there is a period of frequent, intense hot flushes and then months of mild or no symptoms at all. Some women never experience hot flushes, which may reflect a stable serum level of estradiol in their fourties and fifties.

Sleep Issues: Insomnia, Decreased Quality of Sleep

Women describe an increase in sleep disturbance and interruption, and a decrease in sleep quality. They experience fatigue during the day and find it hard to perform the activities of the workplace and family life, or experience difficulty driving and focusing.

Women may experience a longer latency to sleep. Falling asleep should take around 15 min in good health. Longer latency to sleep might be defined as taking closer 30 min to fall asleep.

Urogenital Symptoms

Women will experience and report a wide range of vaginal and urogenital symptoms, many of which are treated topically with estrogen products applied to the vaginal mucosa.

Symptoms include:

- Vaginal mucosal dryness
- Vulvar tissue becomes paler and atrophic
- Decreased vaginal secretions and loss of natural lubrication
- Vulvovaginal irritation and friability
- Dyspareunia
- Recurrent cystitis, dysuria
- Urinary urgency, urinary incontinence
- Decreased libido and sexual sensation, orgasm quality, or ability to achieve orgasm

Mood and Cognition

In my practice and research, I have found that cognitive issues, especially in perimenopause, are more prevalent than has been assumed. In the past, clinicians have not been prone to ask questions about cognitive fuzziness and memory loss, and that women have not necessarily connected these experiences, which they find very frustrating, with changes of perimenopause. More women work in challenging jobs than ever before, and their rise up the ladder happens during the perimenopausal and menopausal years. Many of these women will identify cognitive fuzziness and short-term memory loss as the primary menopausal symptom they want relief from, as they need to be fully functioning in the workplace.

Women describe mood and cognitive changes such as depressed or anxious mood, irritability, and moodiness that are not related to external issues. Increased depression and anxiety may be superimposed on chronic mood disorders, but more commonly, women report that these symptoms are not typical. Disruption of neurobiological actions of estradiol and progesterone is consistent with mood and cognitive issues. It is important to remember that sleep disruption may precipitate or exacerbate mood and cognitive changes. The symptoms usually appear gradually.

Patients Experience and Report Cognitive Problems in the Following Ways

- Decreased ability to concentrate and focus
- Less attentive and easily distracted
- Decreased short-term memory
- Decreased verbal fluency, including.
  - Difficulty completing sentences
  - Losing train of thought
  - Difficulty with word finding
  - Difficulty remembering names

Bibliography

1. Archer DF, Sturdee DW, Baber R, et al. Menopausal hot flushes and night sweats: where are we now? Climacteric. 2011;14(5):515–28.
2. Berent-Spillson A, Persad CC, Love T, et al. Hormonal environment affects cognition independent of age during the menopause transition. J Clin Endocrin Metab. 2012;97(9):E1686–94.
3. Beyer C, Rune G. Steroids in the brain: regulators of brain plasticity and protectors against neuronal damage. J Steroid Biochem Mol Biol. 2012;131:1.
4. Craig MC, Murphy DG. Oestrogen, cognition and the maturing female brain. J Neuroendocrinol. 2006;19:1–6.
5. Dumas J, Salerno J, Newhouse P. The role of estrogen in the development of age-related cognitive impairment and dementia. Psychiatric Times. 1 Apr 2006; p. 34.
6. Sartori MGF, Feldner PC, Jarmy-Di Bella ZIK, et al. Sexual steroids in urogynecology. Climacteric. 2011;14:5–14.
7. Tan O, Bradshaw K, Carr BR. Management of vulvovaginal atrophy-related sexual dysfunction in postmenopausal women: an up-to-date review. Menopause. 2012;19(1): 109–17.

5. FAQ: Bioidentical Hormones: Compounded and Non-compounded

Keywords Bioidentical hormones • Vivelle • Suzanne Somers • Estradiol • Progesterone

Introduction

There's a great deal of confusion about what bioidentical hormones are, how they relate to once-standard prescriptions like Premarin, and whether they are natural or synthetic or organic. Additional confusions circle around whether bioidentical HT hormones have to be compounded at a special compounding pharmacy, whether that is a safe practice, and whether bioidentical hormones are available through ordinary prescription of FDA-regulated and manufactured hormone products.

Q. What are bioidentical hormones?

A. Traditionally, estrogen has been delivered as HT in the form of conjugated equine estrogen (CEE/brand name Premarin, Cenestin), a form of estrogen derived from female horse urine, and taken orally. Oral estrogen has also been produced as an estropipate, derived from plant source, and manufactured from purified crystalline estrone (brand names Ogen and Ortho-Est). Esterified Estrogen has been derived from soy and wild yams (brand names: Estratab, Menest) and combines several estrogens. Table 5.1 lists the synthetic sources of bioidentical hormones; Table 5.2 lists bioidentical hormone derived from natural or semi-synthetic sources.

CEE and other nonbioidentical estrogens are similar to human estrogen, but are not an exact match, hence the description of these more exactly matching hormones as bioidentical. Bioidentical hormones are made to exactly match human hormone, and the drugs are micronized into superfine hormone particle for increased absorption.

K. Sherif, *Hormone Therapy: A Clinical Handbook*,
DOI 10.1007/978-1-4614-6268-2_5,

Table 5.1. Bioidentical hormone from synthetic sources.

Estrace
Gynediol
Estraderm
Vivelle
Climara
Fempatch
Esclim
Prometrium

Table 5.2. Bioidentical hormone from natural or semi-synthetic sources.

Triest
Biest
Estrone
Estradiol
Estriol
Progesterone
DHEA
Testosterone

The argument has been that in the cascading action of steroid hormones, an inexact match negates some of the possible effect of CEE, and that bioidentical estrogen and other hormones offer better relief, because they flow better, connect better with hormone receptors, and fit more seamlessly into the endocrinal system.

The debate over bioidentical estrogens has little to do with whether the estrogen is created synthetically in a lab, or manufactured from an animal source. The interest in bioidentical hormones is in treating the body with specific ratios of the different kinds of estrogens that the body would produce, and in introducing into the body the precise chemical compound of estrogen that the body would have produced by itself.

Bioidentical estrogens are not natural per se, though they are derived from plant source. These products are made from diosgenin, which is a plant oil extracted from soybeans and from wild yams. In the lab, it is altered chemically to become an exact match to human hormone. As a natural source, bioidentical hormone cannot be patented (human hormones, too, are not patentable, which is why the drug companies have created replacement hormones with a slight difference from the human version). What pharmaceutical companies patent on bioidentical HT are the patch delivery systems.

Q. When were bioidentical hormones invented and popularized?

A. Bioidentical hormone derived from diosgenin has been known since the 1930s. The route of administration was incredibly painful: it was injected into the muscle, using an oil-based solution. Interest was aroused in bioidentical hormones after the mid-1970s, in response to the rise of HT-related endometrial cancer, which was responded to by a form of HT that balanced estrogen and progesterone. This resulted in the creation of the synthetic progesterone -- progestin -- and the concept of opposed therapy. By the late 1980s, lab scientists were able to micronize the hormones, producing drugs with ultra-fine particles that are more readily absorbed. This raised the absorption rate of oral progesterone. It made possible the use of micronized estradiol using a transdermal route. Micronized progesterone was approved by the FDA in 1998.

Q. What are the two kinds of bioidentical hormones?

A. The first kind is standardized bioidentical hormone, commercially produced by pharmaceutical companies, under FDA approval for the medicines and the preparation.

The second kind is compounded bioidentical hormones, also made from FDA-approved medicines, but are clinician-prescribed and then produced specifically by a pharmacist who specialized in compounding.

Q. What are the FDA-approved bioidentical hormones?

A. Table 5.3 shows the standardized bioidentical hormones.

Q. For combined/opposed therapy, is bioidentical estrogen and progesterone available together?

A. Not at this time. The drug companies have not yet produced a patch that combines both hormones in bioidentical form. Women with an intact uterus will need a second prescription for bioidentical progesterone, or will need to use a drug formula made of bioidentical estrogen and nonbioidentical progestin, as above.

Q. What are compounded bioidentical hormones?

A. Compounded bioidentical hormones are individually mixed by a compounding pharmacist to meet the clinician's exact specifications

Table. 5.3. Routing/regimen and brand names.

Routing/regimen	Brand name
Estradiol transdermal patch	Vivelle, Climara, Estraderm, Alora
Estradiol transdermal gel	Estrogel, Elestrin, Divigel
Estradiol transdermal cream	Estrasorb
Estradiol vaginal	Estring (vaginal ring), Estrace (cream), Femring, Vagifem (vaginal tablet)
Estradiol oral	Estrace
Estradiol transdermal spray	Evamist
Progesterone vaginal gel	Prochieve 4 %
Progesterone oral	Prometrium
Estrogen/progesterone combined transdermal (bioidentical estrogen/nonbioidentical progestin)	CombiPatch (17-beta estradiol and norethindrone acetate)
Estrogen/progesterone combined transdermal (bioidentical estrogen/ nonbioidenticalprogestin)	Climara Pro (17-beta estradiol and levonorgestrel)
Estrogen/progesterone combined oral	Prefest (17-beta estradiol and norgestimate)

of estrogens (estrone, estradiol, estriol), and progesterone, using whichever route of transmission the clinician prefers (gel, cream, etc.). The prescription can be prepared into lozenges, but these require higher hormone levels and are metabolized through the liver, resulting in similar risk effects as other oral HT, unless very carefully sucked into the inner cheek tissue and not swallowed.

Q. Why do some women and clinicians prefer compounded bioidentical hormones?

A. Using bioidentical hormones, if a clinician and patient wish, the different forms of estrogen (estrone, estradiol, estriol) can be tested, and then replaced in specific amounts to return to more comfortable levels.

Compounding may be helpful to patients who need a dosage in between what brand name preparations offer, especially when balancing estrogen and progesterone levels to maximize efficacy and minimize side effects.

Some patients are allergic to the glue in the commercial estradiol patches or to the oil used in oral progesterone, and these are additional reasons to source medicine from a compounding pharmacy.

Table 5.4. Bioidentical hormones: misconceptions and facts.

Misconception	Fact
Bioidentical hormones are natural	Bioidentical refers to structure; natural refers to source
Bioidentical hormones are custom-compounded	Custom-compounding is one way to obtain bioidentical hormones. FDA-approved drugs are another
Bioidentical hormones are safe hormones	All hormones can cause side effects. A "completely safe" hormone does not exist
Conventional/traditional hormones are synthetic hormones	Conventional hormones may be synthetic or bioidentical. The choice of prescription depends on patient and physician preferences

Source: Sood et al., 2011; Pattimakiel and Thacker, 2011.

Table 5.4 lists the misconceptions and facts of bioidentical hormones.

Q. What is a compounding pharmacy/pharmacist?

A. Compounding pharmacists are specially trained to mix individually specific medicines. These pharmacists are state-licensed and regulated to provide alternatives to off-the-shelf prescription/FDA-approved medicines. They have the education and equipment that allows them to mix patient-specific medicine according to clinician prescription. The medicines they use are purchased from labs and distributors that are FDA-registered and compliant. Compounding pharmacies are used, in non-HT situations, when a patient is allergic to something in the commercially prepared delivery system, or by patients who need medicines used by relatively small patient populations which are no longer profitable for the pharmaceutical companies to produce. Compounding pharmacies are also used by veterinarians.

Q. Is compounded HT FDA-approved?

A. The hormones themselves are FDA-approved. The compounding pharmacist fills the individualized dose prescription; thus each customized dosage is made from FDA-approved medicines, but as an individual product, the resulting compound is not FDA-approved, as the FDS only approved standardized medicine products.

Q. If my patients want or need compounded bioidentical hormones, where can I find a compounding pharmacy/pharmacist?

A. The following are directions for finding a compounding Pharmacy/Pharmacist in your area.

Table 5.5. Estrogen types and abbreviations.

Estrogen type	Abbreviation
Estrone	E_1
Estradiol	E_2
Estriol	E_3
A fourth estrogen is produced during pregnancy:	
Estetrol	E_4

Please see Chap. 1 for more information about the different types of estrogen.

1. Go to web page of the International Academy of Compounding Pharmacists (IACP), http://www.iacprx.org. (An alternate is to use the website of the Pharmaceutical Compounding Accreditation Board (PCAB).
2. That page has a button that says "Find a Compounding Pharmacist." Click on that.
3. Find the button that says "Find a pharmacist."
4. A new screen will come up. It asks you to enter your zip code and a mile radius to search in (5, 10, 25, 50, 100). Depending where you are, you may need to enter a slightly higher mile radius to find a compounding pharmacy.
5. The website offers a telephone number for the locator service. When this book went to press, that number was 1.800.927.4227, though that may change in future years.

Q. How do I prescribe bioidentical HT?

A. Please turn to the "Breakthrough Bleeding" section of Chap. 10: Prescribing Compounded Bioidentical Hormones.

Q. What are the forms of estrogen that are broken down in bioidentical hormones?

A. There are three primary types of naturally occurring estrogens in the human female, as shown in Table 5.5. The relative proportion of estrogens differs between women, especially during the menopausal transition.

Q. Why are bioidentical hormones called "natural" HT?

A. The bioidentical hormones are often called natural, which is somewhat of a misnomer. To clarify, it is not that they come directly and without laboratory preparation, any more than CEE does. Both bioidentical and nonbioidentical hormones are semi-natural and semi-synthetic. It is that the chemical compounds of estrogen and progesterone are exact fits to the body's hormone, whereas the nonbioidentical hormones are slightly different versions of estrogen and progesterone than what the body produces.

Bioidentical hormones are extracted from plants and manufactured in the lab into iso-molecular compounds, which are used by pharmaceutical companies to produce proprietary compounds or proprietary delivery vehicles. Estradiol, estrone, estriol, and progesterone are also supplied to compounding pharmacies.

To the argument that bioidentical hormones provide precise formulations to match the body's own hormone, those critical of them point to errors in dosing possibly introduced by the compounding process. Supporters of compounded prescription return the argument by pointing again to the efficacy of hormones that can efficiently bind to the hormone receptors, thus improving treatment. A compounding pharmacy, for example, can take estradiol powder, mix it into a cream vehicle, and put it into a capsule. Questions of exact accuracy of dosage are less important than the quality of the cream, and whether the cream is fully absorbable.

Q. What is this Suzanne Somers designer bioidentical hormone thing? Is it medically sound?

A. Suzanne Somers' approach typifies the designer hormone therapy phenomenon. The endocrinology behind the trend is sound. In medical practice, we tend to prescribe one dose universally; it makes sense to try to individualize therapy. A typical compounded formulation may combine estradiol, estriol (and sometimes estrone), and progesterone in a cream applied to the skin via a syringe. I have prescribed compounded hormones and have found inconsistent absorption based upon measurement of serum concentrations of sex hormones. The inconsistent absorption is probably based upon the excipient(s) and solubility of the hormone. I usually adjust hormones based upon symptoms. On the other hand, Dr. Morris Notelovitz, whose pioneering innovations are based upon his work of the molecular biology of sex steroid metabolism, uses serum biomarkers to monitor treatment.

Q. How is the designer estrogen phenomenon related to clinicians who prescribe commercially prepared bioidentical estradiol in patch form?

A. Clinicians who prefer conventional bioidentical hormones for HT tend to prescribe estradiol and progesterone in pharmaceutically produced bioidentical formulations. The designer estrogen format might include estradiol and progesterone, but also make use of amounts of the other estrogens, as well as testosterone and DHEA. With conventional treatments, hormone doses are adjusted based upon symptoms. Clinicians who prescribe compounded hormones usually choose doses based upon measurement of serum sex hormone levels as well as symptoms.

Q. What are the positions of the major medical associations on bioidentical HT?

A. The American Congress of Obstetricians and Gynecologists: http://www.acog.org/Resources_And_Publications/Committee_Opinions/Committee_on_Gynecologic_Practice/Compounded_Bioidentical_Hormones

The North American Menopause Society (NAMS): http://www.menopause.org/bioidentical.aspx

The Endocrine Society: http://www.endo-society.org/advocacy/policy/upload/BH_position_Statement_final_10_25_06_w_Header.pdf

Bibliography

1. Files JA, Ko MG, Pruthi S. Bioidentical hormone therapy: concise review for clinicians. Mayo Clin Proc. 2011;86(7):673–80.
2. Pal L. Progesterone: a "weight watcher's pill" for reproductively aging women [editorial]. Menopause. 2006;13(2):166.
3. Somers, S. Ageless: The truth about bioidentical harmones. Three Rivers Press, 2007.
4. Sood R, MD, Shuste Lr, Smith R, Vincent A, Jatoi A. Counseling Postmenopausal Women about Bioidentical Hormones: Ten Discussion Points for Practicing Physicians. J Am Board Fam Med 2011;24:202–210.
5. Wright JV. Bio-identical steroid hormone replacement: selected observations from 23 years of clinical and laboratory practice. Ann N Y Acad Sci. 2005;1057:506–24.
6. Pattimakiel L, Thacker HL. Bioidentical hormone therapy: Clarifying the misconceptions Cleveland Clinic Journal of Medicine 2011;78(12):829–836.

Part II
Prescription of HT

Overview

This section begins with several principles for the practice of prescribing HT, followed by easily accessible information for writing specific HT prescriptions.

- Prescribe to alleviate direct symptoms of perimenopause and postmenopause: the vasomotor symptoms of hot flushes/night sweats, cognitive fuzziness and memory loss, vaginal dryness, and sleep disturbance.
- While commonly prescribed conjugated equine estrogens are effective in treating menopausal symptoms, 17-beta estradiol, prescribed transdermally, is to be preferred, as it is equally efficacious and avoids hepatic first-pass metabolism.
- Route of administration, hormone, and dose matter. As a point of reference, the handbook lists preferred prescribing regimens and gives examples. From that starting point, clinicians can develop regimens with which they are comfortable.

6. Transdermal Estrogen as Preferred Prescription for Perimenopausal Symptom Relief, and the Role of Progesterone

Keywords Transdermal estrogen • Menopause symptoms • Prescription • Compounded hormones • Compounding pharmacy • Patches

Transdermal Estradiol

In light of the history of estrogen use and the studies of HT, up to and especially the Women's Health Initiative (2002) results regarding orally administered HT, the prescription of transdermal HT combines the most efficacious use of estrogen replacement with the safest route of administration, and when prescribed to treat an individual woman's menopause symptoms using bio-identical hormones, is the new gold standard for menopausal hormone replacement therapy.

The transdermal route of administration of estradiol is preferred for the following reasons:

1. Transdermal estradiol does not undergo hepatic first-pass metabolism, avoiding the risks associated with oral route of administration.
2. Transdermal formulations include patches, gel, cream, and spray and are easy to titrate.
3. Transdermal estradiol is associated with a lower risk for venous thromboembolism.

K. Sherif, *Hormone Therapy: A Clinical Handbook*,
DOI 10.1007/978-1-4614-6268-2_6,

Contraindications for HT

Patients already taking HT may develop contraindications while on HT, and HT should be adjusted accordingly, or discontinued. See also FDA Contraindications for HT, chapter 3.

- Breast cancer
- Endometrial cancer
- Venous thromboembolism
- Heart disease
- High blood pressure
- Diabetes
- Acute liver disease (especially for oral)
- Fibroids
- Thyroid disease

The Case for Transdermal Estrogen: The ESTHER Study, 2007

The Estrogen and Thromboembolism Study (ESTHER) focused specifically on blood clots. The study included 271 women, ages 45–70 years. The study was done in France, where a significant number of women were already prescribed transdermal HT. It found that:

- Oral HT quadrupled the risk of venous thromboembolism
- Transdermal HT presented minimal risk (RR = 0.9)
- 46 % VTE cases on HT vs. 36 % in control group

With regard to types of progestogen, ESTHER found that the parent compounds make a difference on their activity on various receptors (progesterone, androgen, glucocorticoid, and antimineralcorticoid receptors) and varying effects on lipids, inflammation markers, and thrombosis.

- Progesterone, micronized progesterone, and pregnane derivatives (including medroxyprogesterone acetate): no increased risk
- Norethindrone, norpregnance derivates: increased risk, up to four times
- Dosage amount was not specifically studied in ESTHER, but a lowest-amount possible approach to dosing was suggested

In conclusion: The ESTHER study showed that hormone type and route of delivery make a big difference, and it pointed to transdermal routing as the safest and most effective way to prescribe HT.

Source: Canonico M, Oger E, Plu-Bureau G, Conard J, Meyer G, Lévesque H, Trillot N, Barrellier M-T, Wahl D, Emmerich J, Scarabin P-Y; for the Estrogen and Thromboembolism Risk (ESTHER) Study. Hormone therapy and venous thromboembolism among postmenopausal women: impact of the route of estrogen administration and progestogens: the ESTHER study. Circulation. 2007; 115: 840–845, and http://circ.ahajournals.org/content/115/7/820.full

The KEEPS Study, 2012

The Kronos Early Estrogen Prevention Study (KEEPS) was designed to compare the effect of hormone therapy vs. placebo on cardiovascular outcomes. Participants included 1,000 women aged 45–58 years (mean age 50 years) with average last menstrual period of 7 months who were followed for 11–16 years. The treatment arms included:

- Triphasic estradiol and norethisterone acetate (NETA)
- Oral estradiol 2 mg daily only (hysterectomy)

The combined primary endpoint was death from any cause, heart failure admission, and myocardial infarction.

The study demonstrates that active treatment compared to control resulted in a reduction in death and cardiovascular events. In terms of cancer, stroke, and venous thromboembolic disease, there were no differences between the two active treatment arms, nor the active arms and control. The KEEPS trial confirms the findings of WHI and other trials that women who start hormone therapy at younger ages have no significant adverse effects, and in fact, may be protected, compared to placebo.

Schierbeck LL, Reinmark L, Tofteng CL, Stilgren Lis, Eiken, Mosekilde L, Kober L, Jensen JEB. Effect of hormone replacement therapy on cardiovascular events in recently postmenopausal women: randomized trial. BMJ 2012;345:e6409 [Online October 2012].

Bibliography

1. Bäckström T, Haage D, Löfgren M, et al. Paradoxical effects of GABA-A modulators may explain sex steroid induced negative mood symptoms in some persons. Neuroscience. 2011;191:46–54.
2. Chu MC, Cosper P, Nakhuda GS, Lobo RA. A comparison of oral and transdermal short-term estrogen therapy in postmenopausal women with metabolic syndrome. Fertil Steril. 2006;86:1669–75.
3. Kublickiene K, Luksha L. Gender and the endothelium. Pharmacol Rep. 2008;60: 49–60.
4. Olié V, Canonico M, Scarabin P-V. Postmenopausal hormone therapy and venous thromboembolism. Thromb Res. 2011;127 suppl 3:S26–9.
5. Wharton W, Baker LD, Gleason CE, et al. Short-term hormone therapy with transdermal estradiol improves cognition for postmenopausal women with Alzheimer's disease: results of a randomized controlled trial. J Alzheimers Dis. 2011;26(3): 495–505.
6. Wroolie TE, Kenna HA, Williams KE, et al. Differences in verbal memory performance in postmenopausal women receiving hormone therapy: 17β estradiol versus conjugated equine estrogens. Am J Geriatr Psychiatry. 2011;19:792–802.

7. The Significance of Hormone Routes of Administration

Keywords Hormone replacement prescription • Estrogen • Progesterone • Estradiol • Hot flushes

Introduction

Oral administration had been the most popular form of HT, until the findings of the Women's Health Initiative in 2002. At times, in the form of Premarin, oral HT has been among the top-prescribed drugs in the United States.

As a result of this popularity and the wide perception of the safety of oral HT, very little attention had been paid to other estrogen routes. In 2002 the WHI evaluation of oral estrogen linked it to raised CHD rates and raised breast cancer rates. These findings had the effect of turning the attention of clinicians and researchers to alternate and safer routes of administration, especially to transdermal routes that avoid first-pass liver metabolism, as they hoped to salvage the use of HT drugs to relieve menopause symptoms, while providing higher assurances of drug safety to women patients.

HT should be prescribed transdermally, especially to perimenopausal women seeking relief from symptoms related to hormone fluctuations and not for any generalized or prophylactic effect. Prescribe the patch first, though throughout this section on prescription, information is included about the various routes of administration, including oral.

Routes of Administration

The primary forms of HT routing are oral, vaginal, and transdermal, with some attempts at routes that are subdermal/subcutaneous, transbuccal, nasal, and that use spray/mist.

K. Sherif, *Hormone Therapy: A Clinical Handbook*,
DOI 10.1007/978-1-4614-6268-2_7,

Oral

The most commonly prescribed HT has been through oral administration. While oral administration is safe in terms of cardiovascular and breast cancer risk in women in their 50s, there is an increased risk of venous thromboembolism. The author of this handbook does not routinely use oral HT, even for women who have had hysterectomies.

Vaginal

Vaginal creams, tablets, and rings have long been used to relieve vaginal dryness and other urogenital complaints, including vulvovaginal irritation, dyspareunia, urinary incontinence, decreased vaginal secretions, concern with orgasm quality and other issues related to orgasm, decreased libido, and other complaints. Vaginal route of administration is not associated with risks of heart disease or cancer.

Topical application of estrogen to vulva and vagina are prescribed when vaginal and urogenital symptoms are primary, or in addition to full HT, in order to treat these symptoms without raising the dosage of the transdermal or oral HT.

In the atrophic vaginal and vulvar mucosa, estradiol may initially raise serum concentrations, but as the mucosa thickens, systemic absorption is limited.

Transdermal: Patches, Gel, Creams

Transdermal formulations include gels, creams, pellets, lozenges, and patches.

Estradiol patches vary in concentration from 0.025 to 0.1 mg/day. Patches are applied weekly or biweekly to the trunk or inner extremities (not breasts).

Estradiol gel is dispensed in a pump, which makes it somewhat hard to dose (i.e., difficult to prescribe 1 1/2 pumps of gel). Gels, like creams, emulsions, spray, can be transferred to other people within 2 h of application.

Estradiol cream is dispensed in a syringe, daily dose is usually ½ tsp. Cream can be individualized and compounded by a pharmacist to include specific dose of estradiol, estrone, and estriol, as well as progesterone and testosterone. There has been concern, however, that estrogen from the creams can easily be transferred to nearby adults, pets, and children, with some reports of spayed female dogs going into heat after contact with human estrogen cream on their owners' arms, and female children showing early signs of puberty as a result of near contact. Patients who use estradiol cream should rub it in very well, wait for it to air dry, and apply it to a part of the body that can be covered by clothing, such as the inner thigh.

Less Commonly Prescribed Routes of Administration: Pellets and Estradiol Spray

Subdermal pellets are placed through an incision in the buttocks, lower hips, or lower abdomen by trained physicians. The pellets are compounded and contain varying amounts of estradiol, estrone, and testosterone alone or in combination. They dissolve within 4–6 months. Some clinicians measure serum concentrations to guide dosing. Using serum hormone concentrations to guide dosing may be more helpful in menopausal women where hormones are relatively static as opposed to fluctuating perimenopausal levels.

Disadvantages of pellets:

- Decreased flexibility in adjusting hormones
- Depots may release higher doses initially
- Progesterone must be administered separately orally or transdermally

Transbuccal lozenges/trouches. Compounded estradiol troches are absorbed through the oral mucosa and taken daily.

Disadvantages include:

- Headaches
- Nasal congestion
- Difficulty dissolving

Evamist estradiol spray is sprayed once daily to the inner forearm.

In October 2010, the FDA issued a warning against Evamist transdermal spray, due to the possibility of exposure to children, nearby adults, and pets, Some daughters of HT spray users were experiencing early nipple swelling and breast development. Some sons of HT spray users had breast enlargement. The FDA did not ban the spray, but warned that women who spray Evamist on their forearms should wear long sleeves to cover the spray. For more information, please see http://www.ncbi.nlm.nih.gov/pubmedhealth/PMH0000324/.

Table of Routes of Administration and Brand Name Drugs

The following Table 7.1 compares routes of administration.

Table 7.1. Comparison table/routes of administration.

Oral	Premarin Estrace Ogen Ortho-Est Estratab Menest Celestin PremPro PremPhase Fern HT Ortho-Prefest Activella	Linked to higher risk of breast cancer and heart disease
Transdermal	Climara Alora Esclim Vivelle Estraderm CombiPatch Compounded	Linked to lower risks for breast cancer and heart disease. Convenience of changing patch once or twice weekly
Vaginal/transmucomal	Premarin cream Estrace Ogen Vagifem Estring Ortho-Dienestrol Compounded	Convenient. Treats symptoms locally, without raised rates of cancer and heart disease
Subdermal/Pellets	Compounded	Convenient. Linked to lower rates of breast cancer and heart disease Cons: incision and local anesthesia. May be hard to find an experienced doctor or clinic
Transbuccal	Compounded	May be difficult to properly ingest through sucking/saliva, and not by swallowing

Bibliography

1. Bäckström T, Haage D, Löfgren M, et al. Paradoxical effects of GABA-A modulators may explain sex steroid induced negative mood symptoms in some persons. Neuroscience. 2011;191:46–54.
2. Cagnacci A, De Toni A, Caretto S, et al. Cyclic progestin administration increases energy expenditure and decreases body fat mass in perimenopausal women. Menopause. 2006;13(2):197–201.
3. Caufriez A, Leproult R, L'Hermite-Balériaux M, et al. Progesterone prevents sleep disturbances and modulates GH, TSH, and melatonin secretion in postmenopausal women. J Clin Endocrinol Metab. 2011;96(4):E614–23.
4. Cavallini A, Dinaro E, Giocolano A, et al. Estrogen receptor (ER) and ER-related receptor expression in normal and atrophic human vagina. Maturitas. 2008;59: 219–25.
5. Cummings JA, Brizendine L. Comparison of physical and emotional side effects of progesterone or medroxyprogesterone in early postmenopausal women. Menopause. 2002;9(4):253–63.
6. Dayspring T, Pokrywka G. Pharmacotherapeutic decisions in menopausal women with cardiovascular risk. Future Lipidol. 2007;2(2):197–210.
7. Empson JAC, Purdie DW. Effects of sex steroids on sleep. Ann Med. 1999;31:141–5.
8. Hachul H, Bittencourt LRA, Andersen ML, et al. Effects of hormone therapy with estrogen and/or progesterone on sleep pattern in postmenopausal women. Int J Gynaecol Obstet. 2008;103:207–12.
9. Laliberté F, Dea K, Sheng Duh M, et al. Does the route of administration for estrogen hormone therapy impact the risk of venous thromboembolism? Estradiol transdermal system versus oral estrogen-only hormone therapy. Menopause. 2011;18(10): 1052–9.
10. Krychman ML. Vaginal estrogens for the treatment of dyspareunia [review]. J Sex Med. 2011;8:666–74.
11. North American Menopause Society. Hormone products for postmenopausal use in the United States and Canada. Mayfield Heights, OH: North American Menopause Society; 2011.
12. Robinson D, Cardozo L. Estrogens and the lower urinary tract. Neurourol Urodyn. 2011;30(5):754–7.
13. Shoupe D. Individualizing hormone therapy to minimize risk: accurate assessment of risks and benefits. Womens Health (Lond Engl). 2011;7(4):475–85.
14. Shufelt CL, Delia Johnson B, Berga SL, et al. Timing of hormone therapy, type of menopause, and coronary disease in women: data from the National Heart, Lung, and Blood Institute–sponsored Women's Ischemia Syndrome Evaluation. Menopause. 2011;18(9):943–50.
15. Skouby SO, Jespersen J. Progestins in HRT: sufferance or desire? [review]. Maturitas. 2009;62:371–5.

8. Hormone Therapy: Individualizing Treatment Based Upon Perimenopausal Symptoms

Keywords Oral estrogen • Transdermal estrogen • Vaginal estrogen creams • Transdermal estrogen patches • Routes of hormone replacement administration

Introduction

All FDA-approved systemic estrogen formulations relieve hot flushes. However, menopausal symptoms are not always equivalent to estrogen deficiency. Women in their 40s have varying estradiol levels based upon BMI, ethnicity and other factors. *I believe that progesterone has an important role in treating menopausal symptoms and balancing estradiol.* Symptoms of high estradiol, such as breast tenderness and enlargement, increased irritability, and frequent awakening (without night sweats), may be best treated with progesterone alone. Administration of estradiol to women with already high (or spiking) estradiol levels may also result in weight gain. While guidelines recommend using hormones for the shortest time possible, I do not believe that women should be encouraged to discontinue them if they feel well and desire to continue.

The suggested regimens in this chapter have been developed based upon a combination of biological mechanisms of action, clinical experience, and clinical trials. As more biological mechanisms of action are discovered, therapeutic regimens will continue to be refined. Knowledge about estrogen and progesterone receptor type, number, and tissue distribution, individual differences in enzymes, and many other known and unknown factors will influence treatment.

K. Sherif, *Hormone Therapy: A Clinical Handbook*,
DOI 10.1007/978-1-4614-6268-2_8,

In general, the preferred approach is:

Transdermal estradiol vs. oral estradiol and non-estradiol preparations.

- Oral micronized progesterone* (OMP) vs. progestins.
- Starting low doses: 0.05 mg/day estradiol patch roughly corresponds with estradiol 50 pg/mL serum concentration, which is in the low follicular range in premenopausal women, as in Table 8.1.
- Monitoring symptoms every 2–3 months.
- Adjusting doses based upon symptoms, not sex hormone levels.
- A discussion of discontinuation of hormones in 6–12 months based upon preference.

Women with menopausal symptoms who may become pregnant may benefit from hormonal contraceptive pills.

Table 8.1. Serum estradiol concentrations during menstrual cycle and reproductive stage.

Menstrual cycle phase	Serum estradiol concentrations (pg/mL)
Follicular	40–200
Pre-ovulatory	250–500
Luteal	100–150
Stage of reproduction	
Pre-menarche	40–50
Postmenopausal	<20

Above all, there is no substitute for good physical and mental health. Absence of healthy nutrition, physical activity, and a solid foundation of healthy relationships cannot be treated with hormones.

Typical Prescribing Regimens

1. Perimenopausal with menses
   (a) Estradiol 0.025 mg patch/gel/lotion
   (b) Cyclic oral micronized progesterone 200 mg days 14 through 28
   - If bleeding is irregular
     - Change to micronized progesterone 100 mg continuously
     - Vaginal progesterone days 14–28

2. Perimenopausal or postmenopausal s/p hysterectomy
   (a) Start estradiol 0.025 mg patch/gel/lotion
   (b) If side effects of estradiol develop, such as irritability, tender or enlarged breasts, add micronized progesterone 100 mg continuously

Considerations for Individualization

1. Women with BMI less than 25 may have serum estradiol variations which cycle rapidly and with higher amplitude that may necessitate higher doses of progesterone.
2. It is safe to prescribe oral micronized progesterone to women with hysterectomy who experience symptoms of estrogen dominance.

For Hot Flushes

- Start low-dose transdermal estradiol (weekly or biweekly patches or daily gel/lotion/spray).
- If flushes are not relieved in 1–2 weeks, increase the dose.
- If hot flushes are relieved, but symptoms of high estradiol develop such as breast tenderness or enlargement, increased irritability and difficulty sleeping, add 100 mg OMP nightly.
- If abnormal bleeding develops with progesterone nightly, switch to 200 mg days 14–28 of the calendar month or the menstrual cycle.

For Cognitive Issues and Mood Swings

- If good quality sleep is restored (using either estradiol to reduce nocturnal hot flushes or OMP) there may be improvement in cognition.
- If cognition remains an issue despite good quality sleep, start low-dose estradiol and titrate as above.

Signs of Excess Estradiol Include:
* Breast tenderness and enlargement
* Migraine headache
* Increased irritability

For Low Libido

- Start low-dose transdermal estradiol (weekly or biweekly patches or daily gel/lotion/spray).
- If flushes are not relieved in 1–2 weeks, increase the dose.
- If hot flushes are relieved, but symptoms of high estradiol develop such as breast tenderness or enlargement, increased irritability, and difficulty sleeping, add 100 mg OMP nightly.
- If abnormal bleeding develops with progesterone nightly, switch to 200 mg days 14–28 of the calendar month or the menstrual cycle.

Transdermal Estradiol Formulations for Dosage and Prescription

Table 8.2 lists preferred transdermal estrogens.

Table 8.2. Transdermal Estradiol Formulations.

Estradiol patch			**All: bypass liver**	**For all: Patches may fall off, hypersensitivity reactions, edges may lift**	**For all: Rotate sites weekly, avoid breasts, generics available**
Alora	0.025 mg/day	0.05,0.075, 0.1		Twice weekly	Twice weekly
Climara	0.025 mg/day	0.0375, 0.05, 0.075, 0.1	Very low-dose available at 0.025	Weekly	
Esclim					
Estraderm	0.05 mg/day	0.01 mg/day		Twice weekly	Twice weekly
Menostar	0.014 μg	2–3 patches	Weekly		
Vivelle Vivelle-DOT	0.025 mg/day	0.0375, 0.05, 0.075, 0.1	Very low-dose available at 0.025 Vivelle-Dot small		Twice weekly (Vivelle Dot not available as generic)
Estradiol gel			**For all: dry quickly**	**For all: risk of transfer to another person**	**Morning application; do not wash area for 1 h**
Divigel	0.25 mg	0.5 mg, 1.0 mg	Very low dose available		
Elestrin	0.06 % gel = 1 pump	2 pumps			
Estrogel	0.06 % gel = 1 pump	2 pumps			
Estradiol spray					
Evamist	1.7 % 1 pump daily	2 pumps daily			For multiple sprays—do not overlap
Estradiol emulsion					
Estrasorb	0.025 mg (one packet)	0.05 mg (two packets)			Apply daily to inner thigh, alternate thighs
Compounded estrogens					
Bi-Est	0.625 mg BID (20 % estradiol, 80 % estriol)	0.31 mg BID 1.25 mg BID			
Tri-Est					

For frequent awakening with or without signs of high estradiol (breast tenderness or enlargement):

- Start OMP 100 mg before bedtime.
- If sleep is not improved with 100 mg within 1–2 weeks, increase to 200 mg before bedtime.

For difficulty achieving orgasm:

- If the prepuce is fused over the clitoris due to atrophy, estradiol cream nightly may help, but this may require surgical intervention.

For heavy menstrual bleeding (regular cycles):

- Try OMP 200 mg nightly days 14–28 of the menstrual cycle
- Medroxyprogesterone acetate (MPA) 5 or 10 mg days 14–28 of the menstrual cycle
- Low-dose intravaginal progesterone gel (Crinone® or Prochieve®) days 21–28 of the menstrual cycle

For heavy menstrual bleeding with irregular cycles:

- Try the above measures but use calendar days, instead of menstrual cycle days

For premenstrual symptoms that have returned or are worsening after years of relative stability:

- OMP 100 mg days 14–18 of the cycle
- Trial low-dose estradiol if OMP doesn't help
- In some women, OMP may have an paradoxical effect based upon differences in GABA receptors

Progesterones

The Table 8.3 lists progestogens.

> Although progesterone is preferable to progestins, progestins may be used when bleeding cannot be controlled with oral micronized progesterone.

> Oral micronized progesterone's sedating effects are magnified by a full stomach, alcohol, and drugs with sedating effects such as soporifics, benzodiazepines, and anticholingerics.

Table 8.3. Progesterone and Progestins.

ORAL route of administration	Generic name	Brand name(s)	Doses	Comments
	Micronized progesterone	Prometrium	100 mg, 200 mg	Peanut oil excipient Somnolence increased with alcohol and meals
	Medroxyprogesterone acetate (MPA)	Amen Cycrin Provera	2.5 mg, 5 mg, 10 mg	Metabolism increased with: rifampin, St. John's Wort, carbamazepine, phenytoin, azole antifungals, phenobarbital
	Norethindrone acetate (NETA)	Aygestin	2.5 mg, 5 mg, 10 mg	Metabolism increased with: rifampin, St. John's Wort, carbamazepine, phenytoin, azole antifungals, phenobarbital
VAGINAL route of administration				
	Progesterone	Crinone Procheive	4 %, 8 % every other day	Approved only for assisted reproduction and for secondary amenorrhea
Transdermal route of administration				
Compounded progesterone cream	50 mg topically twice daily	Titrate up as needed	Bypass liver Less somnolence compared to oral micronized progesterone	Absorption variable

If systemic estrogens do not relieve symptoms of vulvar and vaginal atrophy, topical vaginal estradiol may be helpful.

Vaginal estradiol is not absorbed systemically.

Vulvar/Vaginal Discomfort

See Table 8.4 for vulvar discomfort and/or vaginal discomfort due to decreased secretions.

- Estradiol cream, Estring, Femring, or Vagifem tablets
- It is safe to give vaginal estradiol with systemic therapy, but progesterone must be added for women with a uterus. If systemic estrogens do not relieve symptoms of vulvar and vaginal atrophy, topical vaginal estradiol may be helpful.

Table 8.4. Estrogens for Vulvar Discomfort and/or Vaginal Discomfort.

Cream, tablet, or ring	Brand name (drug type)	Dosage
Vaginal ring	Estring (17beta-estradiol) Femring	2 mg (equivalent to 0.75 mg per day/3 months) per day (new ring every 3 months) 0.05 mg per day/3 months 0.10 mg per day/3 months
Tablets	Vagifem (estradiol hemihydrate)	0.025 mg/tablet. First 2 weeks, 1 tablet a day, then 1 tablet twice weekly
Cream	Estrace (17beta-estradiol) Premarin cream (CEE)	0.1 mg per 2 g cream: first 2 weeks, 2 g daily. After, 1–2 g 2–3 times weekly 0.625 mg per 2 g cream. First 2 weeks, 2 g. After, 1–2 g 2–3 times weekly

Reminders:
* Oral micronized progesterone (Prometrium®) has peanut oil in the excipient.
** In some women with gaba-aminobutyric acid receptors (GABA) differences, giving progesterone may result in paradoxical reactions (progesterone or progesterone-type agonists such as benzodiazepines behaving as GABA antagonists).

Table 8.5 lists FDA-approved hormone formulations that include a hormone component that is not bioidentical. They include both transdermal and oral routes of administration. They are generally well-tolerated but are not the preferred formulations.

Table 8.5. FDA-approved hormone formulations, with a component that is not bioidentical.

Regimen	**Brand name**	**Hormone constituents**	**Dosage**	
Transdermal continuous combined	Activella	Estradiol & NETA[a]	1.0 mg/0.5 mg weekly 0.5 mg/0.1 mg weekly	
	Combipatch	Estradiol & NETA[a]	0.05 mg/0.14 mg twice weekly 0.05 mg/0.25 mg twice weekly	
	ClimarPro	Estradiol & levonorgestrel	0.045 mg/0.015 mg weekly	
Oral combined sequential	Premphase	CEE[b] & MPA[c]	0.625 mg CEE daily × 2 weeks 0.625 mg CEE and 5 mg MPA × 2 weeks	
Oral combined continuous	PremPro	CEE & MPA	0.3/1.5 mg 0.45/1.5 mg 0.625/2.5 mg 0.625/5 mg	
Oral estrogen	Premarin	CEE[a]	0.3 mg 0.45 mg 0.625 mg 0.9 mg 1.25 mg	In women without a uterus: daily, or 25 days continuously, and 5 off.

[a]*NETA* norethindrone acetate
[b]*CEE* conjugated equine estrogens
[c]*MPA* medroxyprogesterone acetate

Bibliography

1. Gleason CE, Schmitz TW, Hess T, et al. Hormone effects on fMRI and cognitive measures of encoding: importance of hormone preparation. Neurology. 2006;67: 2039–41.
2. Gruber DM, Huber JC. Tissue specificity: the clinical importance of steroid metabolites in hormone replacement therapy. Maturitas. 2001;37:151–7.
3. L'Hermite ML, Simoncini T, Fuller S, Genazzani AR. Could transdermal estradiol + progesterone be a safer postmenopausal HRT?A review. Maturitas. 2008;60: 185–201.
4. Mather KJ, Norman EG, Prior JC, Elliott T. Preserved forearm endothelial responses with acute exposure to progesterone: a randomized cross-over trial of 17-b estradiol, progesterone, and 17-b estradiol with progesterone in healthy menopausal women. J Clin Endocrinol Metab. 2000;85(12):4644–9.
5. Montplaisir J, Lorrain J, Denesle R, Petit D. Sleep in menopause: differential effects of two forms of hormone replacement therapy. Menopause. 2001;8(1):10–6.
6. Tremollieres F, Brincat M, Erel CT. EMAS position statement: managing menopausal women with a personal or family history of VTE. Maturitas. 2011;69:190–3.

9. FAQ: HT Prescription

Keywords Beginning hormone therapy • Hormone therapy contraindications • Hormone therapy diagnosing • Breast cancer • Hormone therapy side effects

Q. When should HT begin?

A. When a woman patient reports that symptoms such as hot flushes, night sweats, cognitive problems, vulvar and vaginal discomfort, and poor quality sleep are severe enough that they interfere with her quality of life. Often, the symptoms that most interfere are hot flushes and interrupted sleep, and cognitive issues.

Q. What are the contraindications to HT?

A. The contraindications to HT are:

- Pregnancy
- Breastfeeding
- Liver disease
- Breast cancer, past or present
- Endometrial cancer, past or present
- Endometrial hyperplasia
- Vaginal bleeding of indeterminate cause
- Venous thromboembolism (transdermal estradiol is safe)
- Past history of stroke
- Past history of myocardial infarction

Cautions to use include:

- Family history of breast cancer
- Benign breast lumps (fibrocystic breast disease)
- History of endometriosis or endometrial hyperplasia
- History or high risk of blood clots
- Active systemic lupus erythematosus

K. Sherif, *Hormone Therapy: A Clinical Handbook*,
DOI 10.1007/978-1-4614-6268-2_9,

- History or family history of miscarriage
- Obesity (severe obesity)
- Smoking
- Hypertension
- Hypertriglyceridemia
- Diabetes
- Heart failure
- History of liver disease or liver cancer
- History of gallstones
- Migraines
- Renal insufficiency
- Epilepsy
- History of asthma
- Varicose veins
- Angina pectoris
- Porphyria

Q. Do you recommend any specific duration of treatment? Is there a duration of treatment that should not be exceeded?

A. *Professional societies recommend the shortest duration possible.* For some women, HT for less than a year may be enough. After tapering hormone doses by the month, those who become symptomatic may restart if they want. Prospective and observational studies do not demonstrate risk for over 5 years duration in those who started in their 30s and 40s.

Q. In diagnosing, should follicle stimulating hormone (FSH) be checked? What about the comprehensive female hormone panel?

A. In clinical practice, prescribe based primarily on patient report. FSH is not a particularly sensitive or specific marker to perimenopause, and it will be high in menopause. Treatment should not be based on serum concentrations, but on patient symptoms.

Q. Does BMI matter?

A. Yes. The higher the BMI, the higher the levels of adipocyte-produced estrone. Women with high BMI are less like to have hot flushes.

Q. How do I make prescription decisions regarding HT for women who have experienced surgical menopause through oophorectomey or hysterectomy, or who have experienced medical menopause?

A. For surgical menopause:

- Start low-dose estradiol immediately and taper up as needed every 1–2 months.

- Higher doses of estradiol may be needed to treat hot flushes, but symptoms of high estradiol may develop.
- If decreasing the dose of estradiol results in hot flushes, increase to the next dose and add OMP 100 mg nightly.

Q. How do I prescribe for women experiencing early menopause, and what should I be aware of?

A. With early menopause, women can use the same regimen as women with typical menopause.

Q. When in the day should HT be taken?

A.

- Transdermal estradiol patches are applied weekly or biweekly.
- Transdermal estradiol gel/emulsion/spray are applied in the morning.
- Vaginal estradiol is generally used at night.
- Oral micronized progesterone is taken at bedtime.
- A full stomach or alcohol may triple the amount of progesterone that is absorbed and may result in excess drowsiness.

Q. What side effects should I watch for and ask the patient to watch for?

A. The side effects of too much estrogen are headache and tenderness in the breasts. Excess estrogen results in:

- Breast enlargement and/or tenderness
- Increased frequency of migraine headache
- Weight gain
- Nausea

The side effects of excess progesterone include sleepiness, short-term memory loss, and grogginess.

The side effects of too much testosterone include: hair growth, change in voice, acne, and possibly some aggression.

Q. Which drugs have important interactions with estradiol?

A. Increased metabolism of estradiol resulting in lower efficacy:

- Clarithromycin
- Erythromycin
- Ketoconazole
- Itraconazole
- Grapefruit juice
- St. John's wort

Decreased metabolism of estradiol resulting in higher serum concentrations:

- Carbamazepine
- Phenobarbital
- Rifampicin
- St. John's wort

Q. Which drugs interact with oral micronized progesterone?

A. Excess progesterone may result in drowsiness and grogginess upon awakening. Any drugs that have sedative-type properties may cause excess drowsiness with progesterone, including:

- Benzodiazepines
- Cetirizine
- Diphenhydramine
- Narcotic analgesics
- Soporifics such as zolpidem

Part III
Monitoring, Side Effects, Co-existing Conditions, and Ending Treatment

Overview

When prescribing hormone therapy, it is important to discuss:

- Therapeutic effects and possible side effects
- Need to evaluate response in 2–3 months
- More frequent visits if adjustment at 2–3 months, and fewer if doing well. Discussion at annual visit

This section includes information on side effects and breakthrough bleeding, monitoring patients on HT, prescribing HT with co-existing conditions, and directions on ending HT treatment.

10. Hormone Therapy: Monitoring Effects and Side Effects

Keywords Menopause symptoms • Intermenstrual spotting • Low estrogen • High progesterone • Breast tenderness • Breakthrough bleeding

Questions to Ask

Women taking HT may experience symptoms related to estrogen excess. Symptoms include nausea, weight gain, breast tenderness, and enlargement. Other symptoms include premenstrual syndrome and heavier or light menstrual bleeding. Intermenstrual spotting may occur with continuous estradiol and progesterone.

Questions to ask patients when monitoring their HT

- Have the symptoms subsided?
  - Hot flushes: degree and frequency
  - Quality of sleep
  - Cognition: memory, concentration
  - Vaginal secretions
  - Bleeding pattern
- Have symptoms of excess estradiol developed (may vary by BMI, type, and distribution of estrogen receptors)
  - Breast tenderness
  - Increased irritability
  - Onset of migraine-like headaches
  - Worsening of premenstrual symptoms

Have new symptoms related to menopause emerged, i.e., hot flushes/night sweats; sleep quality; mood swings; cognitive distress or memory loss; libido issues, vaginal dryness, and other urogenital issues.

Has the patient been compliant and regular with treatment?

Has the patient experienced frustration with route of administration that suggests using a different form?

What are the bleeding patterns? Are they consistent?

K. Sherif, *Hormone Therapy: A Clinical Handbook*,
DOI 10.1007/978-1-4614-6268-2_10,

Table 10.1. Signs and Symptoms of HT excess and/or deficiency.

Estrogen too low	**Progesterone too high**
Hot flushes/night sweats	PMS-type moodiness
Sleep disruption/low sleep quality	Sleepiness
Moodswings, PMS-type symptoms	General sense of "feeling bad"
Urogenital symptoms like vaginal dryness	Depression
Estrogen too high	
Breast tenderness or pain	
Headache (vascular/migraine)	

Signs and Symptoms of HT Excess and/or Deficiency

The Table 10.1 shows general symptomatic signs of incorrect levels of estrogen and progesterone, so you can identify symptoms that signal overly high or low dosages of estrogen and progesterone, and correct the dosage.

Corrective Treatments

The following Table 10.2, Corrective Treatment to Hormone Therapy problems, details symptomatic problems and the change to dosage and other options that should provide relief.

Breakthrough Bleeding

Bleeding after the first 3 months of HT should be brought to a clinician's attention (unless a woman is taking cyclical combined HT, in which case periods are expected). Bleeding after 3 months can be the effect of cancer, polyps, or premalignant endometrial hyperplasia. Endometrial sampling or biopsy would be needed to rule this out.

In monitoring, when there is too much breakthrough bleeding, clinicians need to rebalance the ratio of estrogen and progesterone.

If bleeding persists after 3 months, the first decision is either to lower estrogen or raise progesterone.

Table 10.2. Corrective treatment to hormone therapy problems.

Problem	Dosage solutions/alternatives	Other options
PMS symptoms/ moodiness	Change to low-dose contraceptive	Increase exercise
	If on cyclical combined therapy, change to low-dose patch, such as Climara 0.025 during the progestin days, extending into the menstrual cycle	Vitamin B6 50–100 mg daily
	Change to oral Micronized progesterone 100–200 mg qhs during the progestin days	Lower sugar and salt intake
Insomnia/sleep quality issues	Take estrogen in morning, to avoid any stimulant qualities. Change progestin to oral Micronized	
Breast tenderness	Restart HT at a lower estrogen dosage, increase slowly	
	Change to a transdermal patch, steadier levels of HT intake	
	Change progestin to norethindrone or to oral Micronized progesterone	
	Add methyltestosterone (HS Estrastest)	
Hot flushes/ night sweats	Double the estrogen dosage for 4–6 months. After, taper estrogen to a patch. Consider adding testosterone	
Breakthrough bleeding	See Chap. 11, Evaluation of Abnormal Menstrual Bleeding	If patient is under 35 years, consider endometrial biopsy
	Consider a progesterone IUD	Perform hysteroscopy and D&C
	Change to cyclical combined or continuous sequential therapy	
Continued cognitive distress/ memory loss/ lack of sharpness	If patient is getting 7–8 hours sleep consistently, increase estradiol stepwise monthly	
Breast cancer risk increases	Stop HT	
	If patient insists on continuing, lower the estrogen dose (0.5 mg estradiol, 0.3 CEE)	
	Stop HT and prescribe Raloxifene	
Vaginal dryness	Add ½ applicator of estrogen cream PV ×2–3 weekly at bedtime	
	Add Estring vaginal ring, once every 3 months	

Adapted from John David Gordon MD et al., Obstetrics, Gynecology and Infertility: Handbook for Clinicians, 6th edition (Scrub Hill Press, 2007)

If progesterone is relatively low (100 mg micronized progesterone, 2.5 mg medroxyprogesterone acetate) and estrogen is at a medium dose (in the range of 1–2 mg estradiol, or 0.625–1.25 mg CEE), then raise the progesterone.

If the progesterone has been raised and the patient is now experiencing irritability and other moodiness, then lower the estrogen level to avoid these progesterone-related side effects. Lower the estrogen to the next available lowest dose, or if compounding, to a slightly lower dose.

If an estrogen/progesterone rebalancing doesn't provide relief, consider switching to a continuous HT regimen.

Clinicians and patients will need to balance the distress over breakthrough bleeding with the control of menopausal symptoms. This can be a real difficulty. In some cases, HT success may depend on the patient living with the minor bleeding as long as her most severe symptoms are abated.

Contraindications

Patients may develop contraindications while on HT, and HT should be represcribed accordingly or discontinued.

- Breast cancer
- Endometrial cancer
- Venous thrombo-embolism
- Heart disease
- High blood pressure
- Diabetes
- Acute liver disease
- Fibroids
- Thyroid disease

Drug Interactions

The following drugs *increase* the metabolism of estradiol:

- Clarithromycin
- Erythromycin
- Ketoconazole

- Itraconazole
- Grapefruit juice

The following drugs *decrease* metabolism of estradiol:

- Carbamazepine
- Phenobarbital
- Rifampicin
- St. John's Wort

Bibliography

1. Campbell Jenkins BW, Addison C, Wilson G, et al. Association of the joint effect of menopause and hormone replacement therapy and cancer in African American women: the Jackson Heart Study. Int J Environ Res Public Health. 2011;8: 2491–504.
2. Canonico M, Plu-Bureau, Scarabin P-V. Progestogens and venous thromboembolism among postmenopausal women using hormone therapy. Maturitas. 2011;70:354–60.
3. Carcaillon L, García-García FJ, Tresguerres JAF, et al. Higher levels of endogenous estradiol are associated with frailty in postmenopausal women from the Toledo Study for Healthy Aging. J Clin Endocrinol Metab. 2012;97(8):2898–906.
4. MacLennan AH. HRT in difficult circumstances: are there any absolute contraindications? Climacteric. 2011;14:409–17.

11. FAQ: Evaluation of Abnormal Menstrual Bleeding

Keywords Endometrial cancer • Breakthrough bleeding • Postmenopausal bleeding • Bleeding on combined HT regiments • HT and periods

Postmenopausal bleeding is the most common symptom of endometrial cancer and always requires work-up. If a woman is using sequential hormone therapy, she may have monthly bleeding, which is expected. Most postmenopausal women using hormone therapy are on continuous regimens and do not have vaginal bleeding. The risk of endometrial cancer is reduced, but not absent, with the addition of progesterone.

Differential Diagnosis

- Most likely in early menopause: Endometrial hyperplasia/ inadequate progesterone.
- Most likely in late menopause: vaginal or uterine atrophy.
- Most common overall:
  - Atrophy (60 %) caused by erosions of atrophied tissues
    - Vaginal atrophy, including erosion by foreign body such as pessary
    - Uterine atrophy
  - Endometrial polyps (10 %)
  - Endometrial carcinoma (10 %)
  - Endometrial hyperplasia (10 %)
    - Inadequate progesterone with estradiol hormone therapy
    - Tamoxifen in women not using hormones
- Less than 1 %
  - Leiomyomata (later menopause)
  - Cervical, ovarian, fallopian malignancy

K. Sherif, *Hormone Therapy: A Clinical Handbook*,
DOI 10.1007/978-1-4614-6268-2_11,

Evaluation

- Endometrial biopsy first followed by transvaginal sonograpy
  - Endometrial biopsy—sensitive for neoplasia, but not polyps or fibroids
  - Transvaginal sonography detects endometrial stripe (should be <3–5 mm depending on specific guidelines), and structural abnormalities in uterus, ovaries, and fallopian tubes. *A thin endometrial stripe does not exclude endometrial carcinoma.*
    - Many patients with negative EMB and thickened EMS will have polyps
  - Other less commonly employed tests include: saline-infusion sonography and hysterography

> A thin endometrial stripe *does not* exclude endometrial carcinoma.

Q. Will a woman who is perimenopausal continue to have periods on HT?

A. Yes. In the first 3 months of starting HT, women may have intermenstrual spotting, especially if she is using continuous progesterone instead of sequential. If this continues beyond 3 months, the recommended practice is either to

1. Decrease the dose of estradiol to the next lowest (using patch, emulsion, or gel that comes in different strengths).
2. Double oral micronized progesterone to 200 mg for days 14–28, or even 400 mg. The risk of 400 mg is grogginess in the morning.

Q. Are there generalizations about bleeding on combined HT regimens?

A. On cyclic/sequential combined regimens, most women will have periods. Although this is most often seen in perimenopause, it can occur in postmenopausal women as well. If the bleeding is bothersome, change to a continuous regimen.

On continuous combined HT, where estrogen and progestogen are taken daily, most women will not experience periods, and the combination results in atrophy of the endometrium. Some spotting or bleeding may occur intermittently during the first month or so.

Q. When is breakthrough bleeding a cause for concern? When should women with breakthrough bleeding be advised to call their clinician?

A. A woman on a cyclic HT regimen, with progestogen taken, will begin to bleed as progestogen is withdrawn. Bleeding at other times, and especially any persistent bleeding, needs to be addressed.

A woman on a continuous combined regimen should expect some bleeding or spotting. She should experience a cessation of periods by 4 months after the start of HT. Any bleeding or spotting that occurs after three or four months of starting should be reported to the clinician and investigated.

Bleeding that continues beyond 3–4 months raises suspicions of a pathological process, including endometrial carcinoma. Women should be counseled to report this bleeding so that it can be evaluated quickly.

12. FAQ: Ending HT

Keywords Ending hormone replacement therapy • HT withdrawal • Menopausal symptoms • Withdrawal before menopause • Withdrawal after menopause

The duration of HT depends on balancing the presence of risk factors and the patient's preferences. Some patients will want to continue indefinitely on HT. Others will want to get the most relief in the shortest amount of time possible.

Q. Is there a suggested duration of hormone therapy?

A. *Patient preference*

A typical scenario would be that a patient starts HT, and returns in about 2–3 months to report how she feels. If she requires an adjustment, she can return in another 2–3 months. After that, she returns for her annual visit (6 months later).

If she is doing well, she may want to continue. If she doesn't think it makes much of a difference, she can stop. If she is on the lowest dose of estradiol and/or progesterone, she does not need to taper. Generally, what is recommended is to taper down estradiol patches one strength, 1 month at a time. If symptoms return, she can increase to the next highest dose.

Clinician preference

Clinicians are in the unique position of knowing the risk/benefit ratio. Several strategies can be suggested regarding continuing or stopping HT treatment:

The most likely situations for discontinuing hormones are

1. The hormones don't seem to make any difference in any symptoms
2. The presence of adverse effects
3. Postmenopausal bleeding

K. Sherif, *Hormone Therapy: A Clinical Handbook*,
DOI 10.1007/978-1-4614-6268-2_12,

The oft-mentioned recommendation for limiting hormones to less than 5 years is based upon the physiology of the perimenopausal transition in which the 3 years before the last menstrual period and the 2 years following it are the years in which there is the most hormone fluctuation. That 5-year window is associated with the most symptoms. However, women may notice an improvement in subtle symptoms that are not as dramatic as hot flushes and may want to continue. These symptoms are not as likely to be based on serum sex steroid fluctuations as they are on the gradual reduction of endogenous hormones after the early menopause.

The surest way to determine if a woman feels well on hormones is to discontinue and monitor for symptoms.

Q. What are clinically proven best practices for withdrawing patients from HT?

A. A slow weaning from HT is preferred, either to end treatment, or while monitoring, to help the patient assess the efficacy of HT.

To withdraw:

If patient is not already on the lowest dose, move down to the lowest dose incrementally and in stages when necessary, and then to nothing.

For oral and transdermal/patches, follow the prescription availability.

For compounded creams and other preparations, decrease by one-half every month.

Patients should be staged for 1 month at the lowest available dose before ending HT altogether.

Q. How long should this process take, from start to finish?

A. It varies depending on how high a dosage the patient was on at the start.

Q. What do patients experience while and after withdrawing from HT?

A. Women withdrawing from HT may experience menopausal symptoms and may have mood changes and difficulty sleeping and hot flushes.

Withdrawal effect: may have mood changes and difficulty sleeping and hot flushes.

- If HT was prescribed to a perimenopausal woman, and the treatment is ended before the woman's natural time of menopause, that woman may start to experience bleeding and periods again.

- If HT is discontinued postmenopausally, there is a chance that a woman may experience bleeding or spotting, lasting as long as two to three weeks after she stopped taking or applying HT. Clinicians should advise patients to call and report if they experience any more bleeding than this.

Q. What if after withdrawing, my patient wants to return to HT?

A. Reevaluate to see whether the woman wants to return to HT, or continue to stay off of it. Clinician must evaluate perceptions of medical risk from the woman's health history along with the patient's desires.

Bibliography

1. LaCroix AZ, Chlebowski RT, Manson JE, et al. Health outcomes after stopping conjugated equine estrogens among postmenopausal women with prior hysterectomy: a randomized controlled trial. JAMA. 2011;305(13):1305–14.

13. FAQ: HT and Other Conditions: Uterine Fibroids, Autoimmune disease, Hypothyroidism, and History of Breast Cancer

Keywords Uterine fibroids • Hypothyroidism • HT and thyroid disease • Hormones and thyroid • HT and antidepressants

Q. Are women with uterine fibroids appropriate candidates for HT?

A. Although uterine fibroids are sensitive to estradiol and progesterone and may be stimulated with the addition of exogenous estradiol, fibroids are NOT a contraindication for HT. HT has been shown to increase the size of fibroids post-menopausally. However, fibroids tend to be less of a clinically significant issue in the late perimenopause when HT is more likely to be started. If fibroids do present a problem with growth and bleeding, the usual course of action is to delay HT until after menopause. Besides levels of endogenous or exogenous sex steroids, there are other factors that affect the behavior of fibroids, including genetics, BMI, inflammation, and environment.

Q. How does HT affect the thyroid?

A. Due to the high prevalence of thyroid disease, especially hypothyroidism, all women should have TSH and free T4 measured annually. The administration of estradiol increases thyroid-binding globulin, which decreases the availability of levothyroxine and triiodothyronine. TSH does not need to be measured after starting HT (except annually) unless a woman becomes symptomatic.

If HT isn't effective, it could be due to thyroid difficulty, and a coexistent hypothyroidism. According to Harvard Medical School's Thyroid Service, by age fifty, nearly one in ten women experience thyroid problems, with these conditions often presenting in women of perimenopausal age. In addition, the transitional quality of perimenopause and menopause can demand more thyroid hormone than the body is

K. Sherif, *Hormone Therapy: A Clinical Handbook*,
DOI 10.1007/978-1-4614-6268-2_13,

used to producing. Some patients have borderline thyroid during their thirties and forties, and with a closer approach to menopause, thyroid function is pushed over the edge into actual low thyroid.

When a woman with borderline to low thyroid takes estrogen replacement, the estrogen increases thyroid-binding globulin in the bloodstream. This gathers and pulls together more thyroid hormone than had been the case. The bound-up thyroid hormone is no longer able to enter cells and do the metabolic work it is supposed to do. It is hard to test for this inactivity: the thyroid hormone is in the bloodstream, just not able to do its proper work, and thus the usual tests for thyroid (T-3 uptake, Total T-4, Total T-3, and TSH) will tend to show up as normal. One possible testing scenario is to order free T-3 and free T-4 blood tests along with a thyroid antibodies test. Any out-of-the-ordinary results on these three tests would suggest a trial prescription of thyroid hormone or non-prescription method of boosting thyroid function. Factors to consider are any prior thyroid irregularity in the patient's history, and the presence of genetic thyroid disease in her family.

This is important to know in relation to HT because the symptoms of menopause are similar to some of the symptoms of low thyroid and Hashimoto's thyroiditis (cognitive fuzziness, irritability, sleep disturbance, and so on). Further, a low thyroid syndrome can magnify menopause symptoms. Relieving the thyroid condition may relieve some of the menopausal symptoms with which it overlapped. This may be enough relief for some patients. If not, getting thyroid function back to normal will at least make it more possible for HT to be effective.

Q. Is HT contraindicated in autoimmune disease?

A. HT is not contraindicated in autoimmune disease, except in one case: active systemic lupus erythematosus.

Q. Are there differences in HT efficacy among women of different ethnic/racial groups?

A. There are no known documented differences in efficacy. There are differences in self-reporting of symptoms and requests for HT information. Women with higher BMI are less likely to experience hot flushes.

Q. How should women with a history of breast cancer with vulvovaginal discomfort and/or dyspareunia be treated?

A. It is safe to prescribe intravaginal estradiol in women with a history of breast cancer, including rings, tablets, and creams. Progesterone does not need to be prescribed to prevent endometrial hyperplasia.

Q. Is HT safe to use in women taking antidepressants?

A. There is no contraindication to HT in women taking antidepressants (except St. John's Wort which decreases the metabolism of estradiol). Too much estradiol can increase irritability. Progesterone may lower mood in some women.

Q. Is HT safe to use in women with history of venous thromboembolism?

A. Only transdermal estradiol is safe, including in women with inherited thrombophilias. Any form of progesterone will not affect VTE risk.

Q. Is HT safe in women taking anticonvulsants?

A. It is not clear if HT is safe in women with seizure disorders. Progesterone (not progestins) is known to increase the seizure threshold, but is not used therapeutically for seizures.

Bibliography

1. Crandall CJ, Guan M, Laughlin GA. Increases in serum estrone sulfate level are associated with increased mammographic density during menopausal hormone therapy. Cancer Epidemiol Biomarkers Prev. 2008;17(7):1674–81.
2. Fournier A, Berrino F, Clavel-Chapelon F. Unequal risks for breast cancer associated with different hormone replacement therapies: results from the E3N cohort study. Breast Cancer Res Treat. 2008;107(1):103–11.
3. Islander U, Jochems C, Lagerquist MK, et al. Estrogens in rheumatoid arthritis; the immune system and bone. Mol Cell Endocrinol. 2011;335:14–29.
4. King J, Harper Wynne C, Assersohn L, Jones A. Hormone replacement therapy and women with premature menopause—a cancer survivorship issue. Eur J Cancer. 2011;47:1623–32.
5. Schwartz E, Holtorf K. Hormone replacement therapy in the geriatric patient: current state of the evidence and questions for the future. Estrogen, progesterone, testosterone, and thyroid hormone augmentation in geriatric clinical practice: part 1. Clin Geriatr Med. 2011;27:541–59.
6. Sjoquist KM, Martyn J, Edmondson RJ, Friedlander ML. The role of hormonal therapy in gynecological cancers—current status and future directions. Int J Gynecol Cancer. 2011;21:1328–33.
7. Ziva Cerne J, Novakovic S, Frkovic-Grazio S, et al. Estrogen metabolism genotypes, use of long-term hormone replacement therapy and risk of postmenopausal breast cancer. Oncol Rep. 2011;26(2):479–85.

Part IV
The Medical and Cultural History of HT

Overview

More than many other fields of medicine, women's health is often rife with controversy. HT has had its share since the late nineteenth century understanding of estrogen and the sex hormones, and the ability to manufacture estrogen from horse urine and synthesize estrogen compound in the lab.

This section provides a narrative of the long history of HT use, its promotion by pharmaceutical companies, and the observational and clinical trials that are often confusing to sort out. Whereas now HT is prescribed specifically around perimenopause and menopause to treat specific symptoms, this was not always the case. The health claims associated with HT have been many, from assuring sexiness to promising wrinkle-free skin and youthfulness forever, even into the 1980s, 90's and 2000s when clinical trials that would shift medical perspectives on safety were being reported.

Both chapters of this section discuss the 2002 findings of the Women's Health Initiative, the controversy around that study design and its findings, and its clinical results.

14. History of HT Use: Controversies and Confusions

Keywords History of estrogen use • Women's Health Initiative • WHI • Breast cancer • Heart disease • Premarin

From its inception, estrogen treatments for menopausal women were conflated with general facets of aging that women experience, with the effect that from the beginning, scientists were interested in estrogen and HT for these broad concerns, and early research, as well as continuing use and promotion, often had a "fountain of youth" quality. Menopause was seen as not just a decline in estrogen, but a general and absolute decline in a woman's attractiveness and quality of life. Her ovaries were described as shriveling with menopause, and that metaphor was also used to describe her postmenopausal quality of life and self-identity.

Over the decades of use, the generalized use of HT vacillated between this element, and a movement away from the decline/attractiveness argument for prescription and toward one that emphasized prevention of diseases of female aging. This has been one reason for the confusion of what HT treats, and even, the confusion around which symptoms are related to menopause and lowered estrogen, and which are not. That is why many sources show a long list of menopause symptoms, many of which are general symptoms of aging, not necessarily related to estrogen deficiency. This has been very confusing to patients.

This history of HT use and controversy is included because it has been very hard for women patients to figure out HT, and even complicated for clinicians to know what to prescribe, given the intense media around and marketing of the science and studies of estrogen, and because the medical understanding of just what it is that estrogen replacement can accomplish has expanded and contracted and done about-turns several

K. Sherif, *Hormone Therapy: A Clinical Handbook*,
DOI 10.1007/978-1-4614-6268-2_14,

times over the past decades. (The author is indebted to Rothenberg 2005 for her overview treatment of the history of hormone therapy in Europe and the United States.)

The First Attempts at Manufacturing Synthetic Estrogen (1880s to World War II)

In 1899, *The Merck Manual of Diagnosis & Therapy* prescribed Ovariin for a woman's *climacterica*, the then-current term for menopause. Ovariin was manufactured from dried and pulverized cow ovaries, as the ovaries were believed to have an estrogen-level raising effect.

Around the same years, Merck & Co was researching and developing the medical use of animal glands. It is worth remembering that at this time and until World War II, the now-large pharmaceuticals were much smaller companies. They produced medicine components. Doctors then purchased these components over the counter and mixed their own medicines for patients. This changed around World War II, when penicillin products (sulfanilamide, and then penicillin and streptomycin) were developed and sold directly by the pharmaceutical companies, with no individual mixing necessary, thus changing the prior relationship, and removing doctors from the business of mixing medicines.

Important strands of this early research into sex hormone replacement saw the therapy as a fountain of youth and were explicit about that. The research also relied in self-experiments, such as that in 1889 by Dr. Charles-Edoaurd Brown-Sequard, a French doctor who injected himself with extracts made from a mixture of guinea pig and dog testicle, and claimed that he felt great after.

The 15 years from 1923 to 1938 was first key period of estrogen research and it featured the work of Dr. Edgar Allen and Dr. Edward Doisy. Allen and Doisy established the role and effects of estrogen and understood the relations between the female hormones. It was at this early date that scientists, pharmacists, and drug manufacturers began to understand estrogen replacement as not only treating specific effects, but also as offering benefit to conditions and possibilities that patients were not yet seeing as problem areas, including unwrinkling skin, birth control, a cure for infertility, an agent for thickening hair that thinned with age, and all issues having to do with menstruation and menopause and aging.

The first commercial estrogen product, Emmenim, was produced in 1930. Emmenim was manufactured from urine collected from women during late pregnancy when E_4 is present. The next source for estrogen supply was the urine of stallions, which have the largest and most potent estrogen supply of all animals. Production focus then shifted to the urine of mares, and then, to pregnant mares, mares being easier to collect the urine from, despite their having less of it than male horses. Still, urine from mares has at least double the potency of human urine/estrogen supply and has continued to be a primary source for the estrogen in HT.

1930s and 1940s: The Development of DES

The next estrogen product was developed in Britain during the 1930s. In contrast to urine collected from live horses, this next estrogen product was lab-produced. It was a synthetic formula of nonsteroidal estrogen called diethylstilbestrol, or DES. It was three times as powerful as natural estrogen products, but immediately, health concerns were expressed. Early data on mice suggested that it caused mammary cancer. The JAMA issued several editorials warning against FDA approval for DES and raised serious concerns about DES's long-term effects. The British scientists who produced the formula for DES had put it in the public domain, following a tradition in British science of not patenting lab-developed drugs. The result is that by 1940, several drug companies were applying for FDA approval of DES, with hopes that the drug would be hugely profitable, as the companies had not had to assume the usual risks and costs of research and development.

Several pharmaceutical companies joined together to create the precursor of a lobbying group for DES/estrogen, this being the first time they had ever done so. They submitted a single application to the FDA for the approval of DES and supported it with a unified campaign.

In 1941, the FDA approved DES for four indications, including the treatment of menopause symptoms and menstruation. Doctors were allowed to use the drug off-label, and started to prescribe DES to prevent miscarriage, a usage that the FDA approved in 1947. Already by 1941, it now seems, scientists knew of a connection between estrogen replacement and cervical cancer.

Prescription of DES for menopause during the 1940s followed the model in which any medical or lifestyle complaint by a postmenopausal women was blamed on menopause and estrogen deficiency. As a framework of practice, the syndromes and diseases of female aging were lumped together as menopausal.

This practice set the stage for doctors to promote estrogen replacement, whether synthetic or equine-based, as a drug therapy that would counter and treat all of these supposedly linked syndromes and diseases. Menopause was newly reimagined as a unified pathology, a disease with multiple attached facets, which could be cured by estrogen/DES replacement. Relatively normal women were defined into the pathology of menopause and treated as such. Menopause was seen as a disease resulting from hormone deficiency, one that endocrinologically speaking is similar to thyroid disease caused by the lack of thyroid hormone, or diabetes' lack of insulin.

1960s: Estrogen Forever and the Promotion of HT to Sustain Youthfulness and Femininity

In the 1960s, drug companies released new ads promoting antidepressants and tranquilizers for menopausal women. These were prescribed in quickly multiplying numbers to women at midlife. Menopause was now understood as a kind of malaise, and treated as such. Though this practice was eventually as widely discredited as it had been popular, it paved the way for the generation-wide prescription of estrogen as the next wave treatment for the malaise of midlife that was seen as accompanying (and which may or may not be caused by) the physiology of menopause.

This was the background to the publication in 1966 of a book by Dr. Robert A. Wilson, with the title *Feminine Forever*. The book used language that most physicians and clinicians today would find distasteful. The author wrote of menopause as a tragedy that leads to the destruction of a woman's character and leads her into a state of living decay. The book promised that estrogen therapy offers a menopausal woman a way to return to feminine attractiveness and youthfulness that had been destroyed by menopause.

Linking menopause with the vanity issues of beauty and aging, Wilson was able to outline a new, cohort-wide reason for prescribing estrogen replacement therapy. *Feminine Forever* was a huge success. Articles based on Dr. Wilson's book appeared in all the women's magazines from 1966 on into the 1970s, and word spread. Wilson began treating large numbers of women with estrogen. The pharmaceutical companies were supportive of Wilson's practice and his foundation. Later in 1966, the FDA criticized Wilson's claims, especially his claim that estrogen was an anti-aging drug.

Ayerst, the drug company then manufacturing Premarin, was a big supporter of Wilson's and helped spread the claim that estrogen offered a way to stay young and attractive and sexy through the menopausal years. The ad campaigns around this usage showed images and suggestions that, once again, most practitioners today would feel uncomfortable with, but which were highly effective. The campaigns successfully linked menopause with fears that an aging woman might lose her husband's interest and see her marriage dissolve, and that estrogen replacement/HT was the solution to these fears.

Classic symptoms of menopause such as hot flushes and night sweats were seen less as bothering the woman who experienced them, and more as something that annoys her husband. Thus, taking HT to treat menopause's vasomotor symptoms was about attending to the husband's needs and is sure to get *both* spouses through menopause.

As this HT usage took off for the menopause years, Ayerst Labs released additional ad campaigns to promote the agenda of lifelong use of estrogen replacement. The estrogen forever campaigns were successful. By 1975, Premarin (CEE) was the fifth most-popular prescription in the United States. By 1992, it would be the top prescription in the US.

The 1970s: Estrogen Replacement and the Link to Uterine/Endometrial Cancer

Already in 1971, a study published in the *New England Journal of Medicine* showed a link between DES and vaginal cancer in the daughters of women who had been prescribed and had taken DES during pregnancy to prevent miscarriage. While not directed at HT per se, the media and public reaction to this announcement was very strong, and DES had been used as one of the estrogens prescribed as HT, sometimes alone, sometimes with progesterone. FDA approval of DES use during pregnancy was rescinded 4 years later. This wasn't HT, but it raised serious concerns about estrogen use and cancer.

During that same year, 1971, the NIH brought together scientists to consider again the use of HT for menopause, in light of the cancer connection. There was particular concern about reported endometrial/uterine abnormalities from HT use. The practical outcome was the protocol to nearly always prescribe estrogen/progesterone combined therapy.

By 1975, scientists and medical researchers were showing the raised risk of cancer from HT use in any part of the body that is estrogen-dependent, to include the genital areas, reproductive organs, and the breasts. The *NEJM* published studies that compared endometrial cancer risk in menopausal-age women who took HT with menopausal-age women who did not, and found that women on HT for 5 years or less showed a five times greater risk than women who were not, and that the risk increased with each subsequent year that a woman used HT.

Prescribing clinicians had varying reactions to the reports, with some stopping their prescription of HT, and others continuing, unconvinced that the full case had been made. In the year 1975–1976, prescriptions of HT declined by 18 %, and from 1967 to 1977, HT prescription declined another 10 %. By 1980, prescriptions were down 50 %. The FDA required that warning labels be added to estrogen packages, describing the links. Ayerst Labs altered the suggested indications for Premarin to the classic symptoms of menopause: hot flushes, night sweats, and vaginal dryness. The wider claims for the drug's efficacy were scaled back.

The year 1976 saw the publication of a study that linked HT to breast cancer. Breast cancer is the primary cancer that women contract, and there had long been a poor prognosis for survival, especially in the 1970s. In 1976, estrogen replacement was linked to breast cancer, and the media attention again soared. One especial concern was that the addition of progesterone—which had been done to lower the rates of endometrial cancer—also acted to raise the risks of breast cancer. Women using combined HT had four times the breast cancer rate when compared to women who did not use HT. Studies linking HT to increased breast cancer risks and rates continued through the 1980s and 1990s, with a particular report in 1989 in the *NEJM* by a Swedish team showing that women using estrogen-only HT had after 9 years of use twice the rate of breast cancer as women who were not using HT; the 1992 follow-up study to the original 1989 study emphasized similar results.

The CDC, in 1991, analyzed the many smaller studies, with the result showing that the raised breast cancer risk in HT use did not start until 5 years of use. The breast cancer risk increase after 15 years of use was 30 % higher and these participants were primarily women who had begun taking HT before menopause. Women with a family history of breast cancer experienced more than a tripling of risk. The CDC report suggested that HT use added around 4,700 cases of breast cancer each years, and that it contributed annually to 1,468 largely preventable deaths.

1980s: The Pendulum Swings Back—HT and the Positive Link to Preventing Osteoporosis

Even as the cancer links were starting to emerge, ad campaigns for HT used celebrities like Patti LaBelle and Lauren Hutton, older actresses and singers who would offer up the message of the HT-induced fountain of youth and attractiveness. By the 1980s and the new linkages, this claim seemed culturally and medically naive. A new reasoning for HT use began to circulate: that HT can protect health-conscious women against diseases like stroke, osteoporosis, colon cancer, Alzheimers disease, and heart disease. The new message was very different from that of *Feminine Forever*'s vision that a woman will feel great and youthful if she takes HT. Instead, it was suggested that the wise woman takes HT not for the putatively selfish reasons of wanting to feel sexy and beautiful, but because HT is good for her health, that it prevents diseases linked with aging, and that it would be health-foolish not to.

This new claim was made possible because of studies published in the mid-1980s that showed a positive link between HT and the prevention of osteoporosis and osteoporotic fracture, and suggesting that estrogen replacement helped build bone and improve bone mineral density. The original studies were on women whose ovaries had been surgically removed with oophorectomy, though the findings were publicized as helping women who experienced surgical menopause as well as natural menopause.

In 1984, an NIH conference seeking consensus on osteoporosis warned against the generalized use of HT—their warning was based on the increased cancer risks—but also said that estrogen therapy was an effective osteoporosis treatment and was perhaps the most effective treatment for osteoporosis prevention. This shift began the remarketing of HT as an important osteoporosis preventative prescription.

In this new swing of the pendulum, the negative of the cancer risks was balanced with the positive benefit of preventing osteoporosis, and the latter was seen to outweigh the former. New advertising and informational campaigns emphasized, or perhaps overemphasized, the connection between the menopausal lowering of estrogen and bone loss and configured bone density as a long-term change, that although women in early menopause are not physically aware of the changes, nonetheless, indicates long-term HT use is indicated.

Two years later in 1986, the drug companies created the National Osteoporosis Foundation. National Osteoporosis Awareness Week was designated by Congress and signed into law by President Ronald Reagan in 1987, to be observed in May, near Mothers Day. That same year, the

FDA reversed its 1976 finding and approved estrogen replacement therapy as a treatment for osteoporosis, along with exercise and a diet rich in calcium.

1980s: The Pendulum Swings Back II: HT and Protection Against Heart Disease—The Nurses' Health Study and the PEPI Trials

After two heavily popularized 1980s trials, the pendulum swung toward advocating for the use of HT to prevent heart disease. This emerged from the Nurses' Health Study, which showed positive relationships between estradiol use and lowered rates and risk for CHD. The study was observational in nature and relied on questionnaires completed by RN's. The correlation between HT and positive CHD was later seen not as causal, but as user effect, that RN's would be more likely than the general population to take note of early signs of heart disease and seek treatment, leading to better outcomes that have nothing to do with their HT regimen.

Nonetheless, at the time, the American College of Physicians issued a statement that women with high risk levels for various kinds of heart disease should consider taking estrogen after menopause. This led to a boon in popularity for HT.

The Nurses' Health Study

The Nurses' Health Study began in 1975 with the intention of studying the effects of long-term oral contraception use, with the aim of understanding its relationship to cancer. Over the course of the study, the purview was expanded to include heart health issues, and because a significant number of the nurses—28,000—used HT, the study became a useful investigation into HT's relationship to breast cancer, stroke, and other heart disease.

The Nurses' Study was an observational trial run by the National Heart, Lung, and Blood Institute (NHLB) that began by seeking health information from 121,700 married registered nurses in eleven states. The nurses observed themselves and filled out questionnaires every 2 years. The Study started in 1976 and the nurses were between ages 30 to 55. Throughout the 22 years of the study, information is available on 116,000

Table 14.1. Results from Nurses' Health study.

Breast cancer	More than 5 years on estrogen plus progestins increases risk More than 10 years on estrogen alone increases risk
Coronary heart disease	Current use among recently menopausal women may reduce the risk of CHD Decreased rates of CHD in Estradiol users (RR=0.56) Decrease in CDH events in low-CHD-risk women (RR=0.53) Lowered mortality from CHD in current and past estradiol users (RR=0.72)
Stroke	No raised risk
Colon cancer	Reduced risk
Hip/fracture	Not examined
Cognitive function	Not examined
Eye disease	Reduces risk of "wet" AMD

of the nurses. Four years later, in 1980, the NIH adds an additional component to fund inquiry into female cardiovascular health. Questionnaires were sent and the date base was updated every 2 years until the study was completed in 2008.

The study design assumed that as nurses they would be more able to accurately record information about their health and habits. The response rate for each 2-year cycle approaches 90 %.

Several results from the Nurses' Study suggested correlations between HT use by postmenopausal women and breast cancer, coronary heart disease/stroke, colon cancer, hip fracture, cognitive function, and eye disease. These are seen in Table 14.1, Results from Nurses' Health Study.

The Nurses' Study was seen as undermining the earlier claim that HT linked to increased breast cancer rates, at least in women who used HT for under 20 years. Women taking HT for more than 20 years saw breast cancer risk rise by 42 %. This was welcomed as reassuring news for women who took HT for much shorter periods of time.

PEPI Trials, 1987

A 3-year clinical trial funded by the NIH, Postmenopausal Estrogen/Progestin Interventions Trial (PEPI) studied the effect of estrogen-based HT on heart disease. It especially investigated lipids and blood clotting. The investigators had suspected that the positive linking of estrogen HT with improved heart health had resulted in part because women with heart disease or heart disease risk were not being prescribed estrogen HT

Table 14.2. PEPI conclusions.

LDL is lowered
Triglycerides are raised
Progesterone interferes with the positive effect that estrogen has on LDL

in the first place. The PEPI results were published in 1995, and the conclusions are listed in Table 14.2.

1990s: Heart Disease and Breast Cancer Risks, and Increasing Popularity of Prescription

Throughout the 1980s, the perceived risks of breast and uterine cancer, and the perceived benefits of heart health protection and osteoporosis prevention were balanced by millions of clinicians and women patients, as they decided whether heart disease or cancer was a larger fear. Though in truth, the Nurses' Study and PEPI showed mixed heart health outcomes, these were hard to evaluate, as the efforts to publicize benefits were overwhelming of the ambivalences in the studies.

In 1990, the FDA approved Premarin as a heart disease preventative, even though no large-scale, randomized clinical trial had been done on this usage. In 1992, the American College of Physicians recommended that all women consider HT as preventive treatment, up to and including several decades worth of HT as they aged. The American College of Obstetrics offered similar guidelines, that for women with no contraindications, such as high breast cancer risk, lifelong HT is appropriate and recommended.

By 1992, Premarin was the most popularly prescribed drug in the US. Twenty percent of postmenopausal women were taking HT, often prescribed by doctors who were focused on the bone and heart disease benefits. As before, HT was prescribed generally, to postmenopausal women as a group, and to women who were white and middle-class.

The HERS Study, 1998

The result of this was the HERS study, the Heart and Estrogen/Progestin Replacement Study, sponsored by Wyeth, of 3,000 women with heart disease, studied for 4 years, randomized into placebo groups and combined estrogen/progesterone. The results, released in 1998, undermined the argument that HT improved heart disease outcomes. The women in the study experienced improved cholesterol rates but the women in the HT group experienced no improvement in heart health when compared to the placebo group, and often experienced worse outcomes. This swung the pendulum away from linking HT with improved heart health, and the American Heart Association issued a warning that women with heart disease not use HT.

HT Linked to Blood Clots, 1996

The risk of blood clots had long been linked to the use of oral contraceptives. HT uses lower levels of estrogen as compared to oral contraceptives, which seemed enough to sidestep concerns about blood clot risk increase. This changed in 1996, when several studies, along with the HERS study, showed that women taking HT experienced a higher risk and incidence of blood clotting/venous thromboembolism/VTE.

The Women's Health Initiative, 2002

Many HT studies were observational. Many were small. Many were non-randomized. NIH director Bernadine Healy wanted a large, randomized study that would put to rest the debates over HT's safety and efficacy in relation to heart disease, osteoporosis, and cancer. The Women's Health Initiative (WHI) was a multi-agency, multi-Institute study of 161,000 women, complete with clinical trials and observational trials.

The WHI study hoped to put to rest the various questions surrounding the risks and benefits of using estrogen HT or estrogen/progestin HT. Because some earlier studies had taken results from women with surgical menopause/hysterectomy/oophorectomy, the WHI was designed to study both women who experienced menopause naturally (and who would be given combined/opposed HT) and women who experienced menopause as a result of a hysterectomy, and would be given estrogen only. The most popularly prescribed drugs — Premarin and Prempro, the Premarin/Provera combination — were given to the control group. Table 14.3 describes the WHI Protocols.

Table 14.3. The WHI study: protocol.

Natural menopause	Surgical menopause
16.608 women	10,739 women
50–79 years; mean age 63.3	
Combined HT:	Estrogen only: 0.625 Premarin
Prempro: 0.625	
Premarin plus 2.5 mg Provera	

By 2000, investigators voiced concerns about safety with regard to heart disease incidence. The women in the HT group, as compared to the placebo group, showed greater incidence for heart attack, blood clots/VTE, and stroke. The study continued, as the numbers of women affected seemed small, statistically speaking. By May 2002, the numbers for women taking combined HT (in the natural menopause group) showed increased incidence of breast cancer was high enough that the NIH's own measures for safety in drug trials had been crossed. The risks were higher than the benefits. Differences in ethnicity, age, and health status did not show differences in outcome.

The WHI was to have continued until 2005. Instead, in 2002, the study on women with natural menopause was stopped immediately, as findings reported no protection against heart disease, an increased risk of stroke, and increased risk of deep vein thrombosis. (The study of women with surgical menopause continued, as these women showed no increase risk, as did a side study on memory.) The WHI results, which are described in Table 14.4, indicate that the CEE/MPA regiment should not be initiated or continued for the primary prevention of cardiac heart disease.

Results from different arms of the study were released over the next few years. The Women's Health Initiative Memory Study (WHIMS) had been set up to evaluate claims that combined HT could prevent Alzheimers in postmenopausal women. In May 2003, the WHIMS reported that the women in the HT group, as compared to placebo, experienced a doubled risk of developing Alzheimers, with reports of 1 additional case per 100 women. A helpful online source for clinical use and patient information is *Women's Health Initiative Frequently Asked Questions about the Women's Health Initiative Memory Study* (*WHIMS*), published in May 2003, and available at http://www.whi.org/faq/faqwhims.php.

The estrogen-only/surgical menopause section of the WHI study had continued after the combined HT segment had been stopped. In 2004, this arm of the WHI was also shut down in response to unacceptable levels of risk. The results, which can be seen in Tables 14.5 and 14.6,

Table 14.4. WHI results.

Disease	Result	Details
Breast cancer	Increase after 4 years By 5.2 years, 25 % increase	RR = 1.24 Nominal 95 % CI = 1.02–1.50
Heart attacks	Increase during first year of use By 5.2 years, 29 % increase	RR = 1.24 Nominal 95 % CI = 1.00–1.54
Strokes	By 5.2 years, 41 % increase	RR = 1.31 Nominal 95 % CI = 1.02–1.68
Blood clots/ VTE	Increases during first 2 years	RR = 2.06 Nominal 95 % CI = 1.57-2.70
Hip fractures/ other fractures	Lowers risk; fractures reduced by 34 %	RR = 0.67 Nominal 95 % CI= 0.47–0.96
Colorectal cancer	After 3 years, reduced by 37 %	RR = 0.61 Nominal 95 % CI= 0.42–0.87
Endometrial cancer	No deaths/no increased risk	

Table 14.5. WHI: estrogen only/women with surgical menopause.

Disease risk	Result
Breast cancer	Stable
Heart disease	Stable
Stroke risk	Raised
Hip fracture	Lowered

Table 14.6. WHI estrogen alone trial: major clinical outcomes for estrogen vs. placebo.

End points (no of cases)	Hazard ratio	95 % CI
CHD (376)	0.91	0.75–1.12
Breast cancer (218)	0.77	0.59–1.01
Stroke (276)	1.39	1.10–1.77
Pulmonary embolism (85)	1.34	0.87–2.06
Colorectal cancer (119)	1.08	0.75–1.55
Hip fracture (102)	0.61	0.41–0.91
Total CVD (1,557)	1.12	0.81–1.07
Total cancer (780)	0.93	0.81–1.07
Total mortality (580)	1.04	0.88–1.22
Global index of risks and benefits summarizing overall effects of treatment	1.01	0.91–1.12

reported that estrogen alone does not raise the risk of breast cancer or heart disease, but it did increase stroke risk. Estrogen did lower hip fracture risk. Based on these results, the WHI suggested that HT should no longer be used for the prevention of any chronic disease, that other, non-estrogen-based drugs should be preferred for the prevention of osteoporosis, and that estrogen should only be used in cases where a woman can't take those other medications.

Post-WHI, Post-2002: Results for Hormone Therapy

In the wake of the WHI announcements, prescriptions and sales of Prempro dropped 74 %. The prescription of HT dropped from roughly 19 million female users in 2002 to 7.6 million in 2004. Media coverage was angry and intense; see for example Gina Kolata & Melody Petersen, Hormone Replacement Study A Shock to the Medical System, N.Y. Times, July 10, 2002.

As a result of the WHI findings, the FDA ordered manufacturers to include black-box warning labels for all estrogen-based products, including creams, patches, and lower dose pills. It restricted the use of estrogen and estrogen/progesterone HT to three indications: hot flushes and vasomotor symptoms, vaginal and vulvar dryness, and osteoporosis, although substitutes were suggested where possible: creams for vaginal dryness issues, and other non-estrogen-based products for osteoporosis. Manufacturers brought to market lower dosages of the combined estrogen pills, which the FDA approved, while still showing concern for unknown side effects at various dosage levels.

The post-2002 indication recommendation is the one now known to most clinicians: the lowest dose for the shortest duration for the individual woman.

At a 2005 NIH State-of-the-Science conference, HT was given a new label to distinguish it from the discredited generalized use of HT: menopause hormonal therapy, or MHT, and to attempt to link it more specifically as a treatment for the relief of particular menopause symptoms. There was an attempt to disentangle the specific symptoms of menopause from the wide array of syndromes, conditions, and diseases of female aging that had been associated with menopause in the prior few decades. It was also hoped that SERMS would be able to treat conditions like osteoporosis that had been directly linked to HT treatment, and that SERMS would offer similar protection but without negative outcomes.

Conclusions

Given the long history of controversy over safety and efficacy, a way forward can be suggested so that women in need of symptomatic help for menopausal symptoms can be treated.

In Spring 2011, JAMA reported, in a study on estrogen use alone, for women who had surgical menopause via hysterectomy, that short-term use of estrogen around menopause does not have the same association with long-term health problems. Estrogen effects are not stored in the body, but dissipate, which explains the lack of long-term negative results.

Building from the recommendation of the least amount for the shortest time possible, I also suggest the usefulness of estrogen replacement in the perimenopausal period for women who want and need it, as perimenopause is only more recently understood as significant, and this usage among younger women was not included in the studies above. The next chapter outlines several of the study limitations of the WHI data, as well as the use of transdermally applied estrogen products, which in the 10 years following the WHI announcements have been shown to be radically safer than the oral estrogens that were studied in the WHI.

Bibliography

1. Committee on Quality Assessment. ACOG criteria set. Ambulatory care criteria set: hormone replacement therapy. Number 23, 1997. Int J Gynecol Obstet 1997;57: 331–2.
2. Hormone replacement therapy. ACOG technical bulletin number 166—April 1992. Hormone replacement therapy. Int J Gynecol 1993;41:194–202.
3. Hsia J, Langer RD, Manson JE, et al. Conjugated equine estrogens and coronary heart disease. Arch Intern Med. 2006;166:357–65.
4. Kurian AW, Clarke CA, Carlson RW. The decline in breast cancer incidence: real or imaginary? Curr Oncol Rep. 2009;11:21–8.
5. Li RH, Gebbie AE, Wong RW, et al. The use of sex hormones in women with rheumatological diseases. Hong Kong Med J. 2011;17:487–91.
6. Noel Bairey Merz C, Shaw LJ, Reis SE, et al. Insights from the NHLBI-sponsored Women's Ischemia Syndrome Evaluation (WISE) study. Part II: gender differences in presentation, diagnosis, and outcome with regard to gender-based pathophysiology of atherosclerosis and macrovascular and microvascular coronary disease. J Am Coll Cardiol 2006;47:21S–9.
7. Rothenberg CJ. The Rise and Fall of Estrogen Therapy: The History of HRT. Harvard Law School 2005.

15. The 2002 Women's Health Initiative Study (WHI): What Did It Prove or Disprove? Future Directions

Keywords WHI • Women's Health Initiative • Breast cancer • Heart disease • Osteoporosis

Introduction

The WHI findings were seen as conclusive by some, were resisted by others, and for a third group, presented an opportunity to bring to the fore the use of transdermal routes of administering HT, which had been used more widely in Europe than in the United States, and which were showing many fewer of the negative effects, primarily because it is not metabolized in the liver, as is oral HT, and because of the use, in the patches, creams and gels, of primarily estradiol.

A 2004 response to the WHI findings argued just this, that the study's flaw was that it had focused only on oral transmission and failed to evaluate routes of transmission that were effective against menopausal symptoms, but without the harmful effects or the oral medication.

Additional Criticisms Included

- The mean age of women in the study was 63 years old, and at an age potentially, when cardiovascular disease process has already begun; many were much older than the usual ages at which HT is begun. This is a study flaw, given that the average age of menopause is 51.3. In particular, this means there are no findings on the specific use of HT for symptom relief in perimenopausal women.
  - 42 % of the women in the study stopped taking the HT drugs at some time
  - 10.7 % of the women in the placebo group initiated HT therapy through their own clinician

K. Sherif, *Hormone Therapy: A Clinical Handbook*,
DOI 10.1007/978-1-4614-6268-2_15,

- 3,444 women in E+P group had been unblended
- During the WHI trial, 248 women in the estrogen plus progesterone group—women who had experienced natural menopause group—had hysterectomies, as did 148 in the placebo group
- The WHI study evaluated the use of only one HT regimen: oral treatment, which is metabolized quite differently from transdermal routes of administration (which avoids first pass metabolization in the liver)
- The WHI study did not evaluate the benefits of HT in the treatment of actual menopausal symptoms

The WHI Study Provided Clarity on the Use of HT in Postmenopausal Women:

1. Risk factors increase after menopause
2. Incidence of cardiovascular disease increases after menopause
3. Premature menopause increases risk
4. Surgical menopause increases risk
5. Diabetes increases risk 3–7 times

The clarity provided by the 2002 reports has allowed women's health practitioners to steer patients away from dangerous practices, or practices that may have a dangerous effect, toward a usage that is efficacious and safe. The findings and subsequent debate were an opportunity to refocus the use of HT on perimenopausal and postmenopausal symptoms. The question for practitioners and researchers is what is currently safest as well as most effective when it comes to patient treatment.

Instead of prescribing menopausal HT generally to treat a range of disease, HT can focus on relieving various menopausal symptoms. Each disease of aging can be treated according to a woman's individual risk factors and with protocols specific to that disease's specialty.

Clarity Was Provided on the Safer Experience of Younger Users of HT

A 2006–2007 re-evaluation of specific strands of the WHI findings provided a refined clarity about the youngest users of HT. For women 50–59, the youngest cohort of the study, and the age group most likely to seek relief from menopausal symptoms, *there was no increase in risks of coronary heart disease*. This was true for both the combined estrogen and estrogen-only arms of the WHI trials.

Conclusions

In light of these conclusions the use of HT dropped off with regard to the hoped-for prevention of heart disease and osteoporosis. In 2007, the American Heart Association produced evidence-based guidelines for the prevention of cardiovascular disease in aging women that emphasized lifestyle changes.

These include:

- Weight control
- Exercise, with a minimum of 60–90 min of moderate activity most days
- Increased physical activity in general
- Alcohol moderation and sodium restriction
- Eating fresh fruits and vegetables and low-fat dairy products
- Cessation of smoking, with the use of counseling, nicotine replacement, or other forms of smoking cessation therapy
- The recommendations offered specific guidance on omega-3 intake, suggesting that women in the postmenopausal stage of life eat oily fish at least twice a week, and that they consider 850–1,000 mg of EPA and DHA in women with heart disease, and 2–4 g for women with high triglycerides
- HT and SERMs are not recommended to prevent heart disease in women

Bibliography

1. Machens K, Schmidt-Gollwitzer K. Issues to debate on the Women's Health Initiative (WHI) study. Hormone replacement therapy: an epidemiological dilemma? Hum Reprod. 2003;18(10):1992–9.
2. Kmietowicz Z. Articles disputing link between HRT and breast cancer are "ridiculous" [news]. BMJ. 2012;344:e513. doi:10.1136/bmj.e513.
3. Morris E, Currie H. The British Menopause Society: next steps 2011 [editorial]. Menopause Int. 2011;17:35–6.
4. North American Menopause Society. NAMS 2011 isoflavones report. The role of soy isoflavones in menopausal health: report of the North American Menopause society/ Wulf H. Utian Translational Science Symposium in Chicago, IL (October 2010). Menopause 2011;18(7):732–53.

5. Rice S, Whitehead SA. Phytoestrogens and breast cancer—promoters or protectors? Endocr Relat Cancer. 2006;13:995–1015.
6. Schwartz E, Holtorf K. Hormones in wellness and disease prevention: common practices, current state of the evidence, and questions for the future. Prim Care. 2008;35(4):669–705.
7. Notelovitz M. The clinical practice impact of the Women's Health Initiative: political vs biological correctness [guest editorial]. Maturitas. 2003;44:3–9.

Appendix: Reference Table of HT Brand Names

This is a full reference table in alphabetical order, of Brand Name drugs used in HT. It is the basis for prescription advice throughout this handbook.

Drug name	Company	Drug type	Route of administration	Usual daily dosages
Activella	Pharmacia	Micronized Estradiol, Norethindrone acetate (NE)	Oral E/P combination	1 mg 17beta-estradiol, 0.5 NE, continuous daily dosing
Alora	Watson	17beta-estradiol	Transdermal patch	0.05, 0.075, 0.1 mg. 2x/week
Cenestin	Duramed/ Solva	Synthetic conjugated estrogens	Oral	0.625, 0.9, 1.25 mg/continuous daily dosing
Climera	Berlex	17beta-estradiol	Transdermal patch	0.025, 0.05, 0.1 mg. One time per week
CombiPatch	Aventis	17beta-estradiol and norethindrone acetate (NE)	Transdermal patch/ combined therapy	0.05 mg 17beta-estradiol and 0.14 mg NE, 0.05 mg 17beta-estradiol and 0.25 mg NE. Twice per week
Esclim	Women First	17beta-estradiol	Transdermal	0.025, 0.0375, 0.05, 0.075, 0.1 mg. Twice per week.
Estrace	Warner-Chilcot	17beta-estradiol (micronized0	Vaginal estrogen therapy (describe more)	0.5 mg, 1 mg daily to start, then 1-3 times per week

(continued)

K. Sherif, *Hormone Therapy: A Clinical Handbook*,
DOI 10.1007/978-1-4614-6268-2,

Drug name	Company	Drug type	Route of administration	Usual daily dosages
Estraderm	Novartis	17beta-estradiol	Transdermal	0.05, 0.1, twice per week
Estratab	Solvay	Esterified estrogens	Oral	0.3, 0.625, 2.5 mg/ continuous daily dosing
Estratest				
Estratest-HS	Solvay	Conjugated equine estrogen and methyltestos-terone (MT)	Oral combined cyclic estrogen/ testosterone therapy	12.5 mg CEE plus 2.5 mg MT; cyclic dosing: 3 week on therapy, 1 week off
Estring	Pharmacia	Estradiol	Vaginal Estrogen Ring	2 mg reservoir; replace every three months
Fem HT	Parke-Davis	Conjugated equine estrogens and medroxyprogester-one acetate (MPA), ethinyl estradiol (EE), and norethindrone acetate (NE)	Oral combined continuous estrogen/ progesterone therapy	5 μg EE plus 1 mg NE; continuous daily dosing
Menest	Monarch	Esterified estrogens	Oral	0.3, 0.625, 1.25, 2.5 mg/cyclic dosing: 3 weeks on therapy, 1 week off
Ogen	Pharmacia	Estropipate	Oral	0.625, 1.25, 2.5 mg/continuous daily dosing or cyclic dosing
Ortho-EST	Women First	Estropipate	Oral	0.625, 1.25, 2.5 mg/ continuous
Ortho-Prefest	Ortho-McNeil	Micronized estradiol and norgestimate	Oral combined estrogen-progestin continuous therapy	1 mg 17beta-estradiol (continu-ous) and 0.09 mg norgetimate (pulsed in 3-day cycles)
Ortho-Dienestrol	Ortho-McNeil	Dienestrol	Vaginal therapy	0.1 mg/gram, daily

(continued)

Drug name	Company	Drug type	Route of administration	Usual daily dosages
Premarin	Wyeth-Ayerst	Conjugated equine estrogens (CEE)	Oral	0.3, 0.45, 0.625, 0.9, 1.25 mg/ continuous daily dosing or cyclic dosing
Premarin Cream	Wyeth-Ayerst	Conjugated equine estrogens	Vaginal therapy	0.625 mg/gram, daily
PremPhase	Wyeth-Ayerst	Conjugated equine estrogens and medroxyprogesterone acetate (MPA), ethinyl estradiol (EE), and norethindrone acetate (NE)	Oral combined cyclic estrogen-progestin therapy	Days 1–14: 0.625 mg CEE Days 15–28: 0.625 mg CEE plus 5 mg MPA
PremPro	Wyeth-Ayerst	Conjugated equine estrogens and medroxyprogesterone acetate (MPA), ethinyl estradiol (EE), and norethindrone acetate (NE)	Oral Combined estrogen-progestin therapy	0.625 mg CEE plus 2.5 MPA, 0.625 mg CEE plus 5 mg MPA
Vagifem	Pharmacia	Estradiol	Vaginal	First 2 weeks: 25 μg tablets daily Then 25 μg tablets two times per week
Vivelle Dot	Novartis	17beta-estradiol	Transdermal patch	0.0375, 0.05, 0.075, 0.1 mg. Two times per week

Adapted from John David Gordon MD et al, Obstetrics, Gynecology and Infertility: Handbook for Clinicians, 6th edition (Scrub Hill Press, 2007)

Index

K. Sherif, *Hormone Therapy: A Clinical Handbook*,
DOI 10.1007/978-1-4614-6268-2,